GIVE UP SWEETS

SIMPLE STEPS ON HOW TO STOP EATING SUGAR AND
BE MORE HEALTHY

G. P. ALEX

CONTENTS

INTRODUCTION

Have you ever thought about what you eat? Not just counting calories—the actual food items that you eat. When was the last time you had some fresh fruits or vegetables on your plate or as a snack? When did you last eat a home-cooked meal instead of some highly processed takeout meal? Do you tend to reach for a prepackaged meal long before making your own fresh salad or sandwich? You are hardly alone in this phenomenon. People are so busy with their jobs, lives, and simply trying to survive day by day they barely have time to see *if* they are eating, much less *what* they are eating. And when you do eat do you know what is in your food? Sure, there are the common macronutrients such as carbohydrates, proteins, and fats, maybe some minerals and vitamins, but that's not all that is in your food.

There is a silent killer that is affecting the lives of people all around the world regardless of their age, nationality, or skin color. It is resulting in diseases such as high blood pressure, insulin resistance, type 2 diabetes, and obesity, just to name a few. Almost no foods are safe from it and you likely have already been consuming vast quantities of it throughout your life. This is something your parents, grandparents, and even your grocery store have been giving you every day of your life. There was even a diet that caused people to eat more of this.

This silent but deadly killer is none other than sugar. You have probably had a relationship with this product since you were a baby, as store-bought baby food and breakfast cereals have added sugar (also known as refined sugar) to help extend shelf life and improve taste. You are not alone in this. Highly processed foods are an easy way out when it comes to quick meals when you are low on time. That is not to say that a treat once in a while is a bad thing, but people are eating more and more processed foods as the years go by due to the convenience.

Sugar is not a new addition to human foods. It has been around for centuries in some form. It has had its hand in shaping not only your body but also the world as it has been a type of medicine, a spice, and even a symbol of royalty. Yet these are not the only things that it has had its hand in. This delightfully sweet addition was an instrument in oppression that has led countless people to become addicted to it and led to many diseases.

It is very easy to blame cane sugar and high fructose corn syrup for the problems associated with sugar but they were hardly the first of the sweet treats humans consumed. Before people were able to cultivate any form of crop it was available in nature. The most frequent of the sugars available to the humans of the past—those that lived in regions not covered by ice—could be found in fruits and honey. In places such as the Americas, there were no honey bees—as these were only introduced in the 17th century to help pollinate crops (Garvey, 2009)—but there were agave plants and trees that provided sweet nectar to this region of the world. It didn't take humans long to figure out that if they wanted to keep this golden treat around that they needed to learn to domesticate these wild bees.

Refined sugar from cane sugar, through the use of a sugar mill, was first documented in India in 100 A.D. Before this, sugar cane was only enjoyed by the people of New Guinea, where it grew naturally. It was 8,000 years before it was refined that people of New Guinea were chewing on this plant to enjoy the sweetness it provided. The first recipe to contain the mention of added sugar, around 400–350 B.C., was found in the book Mahābhāṣya by Patanjali as it was used to sweeten a fermented ginger drink as well as with rice pudding.

It was in 327 B.C. that the Romans and Greeks discovered the sugar in India before bringing it back to their native countries to be used as a medicine to treat a wide variety of illnesses. Yet it was the Arab people—in about 650 A.D.—that became the true masters of not only growing this sweet plant but also refining and cooking it. They were the ones that shaped sugar into a rare delicacy that was meant for only those that were royalty or extremely wealthy. This brought about the creation of marzipan—sugar and ground almonds—which was often showcased in elaborate sugar sculptures which regularly appeared at only the most lavish of dinner parties.

Sugar was spread to the rest of Europe during the crusades but was still considered extremely expensive and only the wealthiest of people were able to afford to try it. This trend continued into the 14th century. Sugar became such a demanded product that during the 15th and 16th centuries slaves were forced to grow cane sugar in the Canary Islands, Brazil, and Hispañiola (modern-day Haiti and the Dominican Republic). Sugar was used in everything from medicine, to spice, to food during this time. Sugar was fast becoming more popular than alcohol in the 1600s due to chocolate, tea, and coffee becoming more prevalent in Europe. All these products demanded some of the sugary goodness.

Sugar became so popular that sugar plantations in Brazil required over half a million African slaves to provide the labor so that they could keep the sugar prices low enough for most people to afford it. It wasn't until the late 18th century that maple syrup was starting to replace sugar as most people who were against slavery were trying to avoid the slave-grown sugar. Sadly, the trend of using slaves to grow sugar continued well into the 19th century. In Europe, beet sugar was taking over from cane sugar thanks to a sugar beet variety invented by a French seed company called Vilmorin which not only had a high sucrose content but also allowed for better extraction of this sugar. Sugar was now readily available to everyone at affordable prices and it could be found in almost all homes.

From 1942 to 1966 there was a movement by medical professionals to encourage people to lower their sugar intake as it was not as necessary to a person's diet as other nutrients were. It was noted that there was a correlation between the consumption of sugar and rising rates of obesity and diabetes. This caused people to look for alternatives to their sugar usage. Yet, in 1980, the Food and Drug Administration (FDA) started demonizing fat instead of sugar and the fat-free fad was born. This diet encouraged people to eat and buy products that contained less fat. However, many of these products contained high levels of sugar and so the sugar-related health issues continued to rise and this is where we are today.

Sugar can't be that bad, can it? Well in moderation, no, it isn't, but sadly many people do not consume this product in moderation, either knowingly or unknowingly. Roughly 75% of most Americans are eating excess amounts of sugar and many of these people are actually addicted to sugar. Yes; you can and do become addicted to sugar. By consuming sugar your brain releases chemicals that are similar to those released when partaking in illegal drugs. Do this long enough and the brain starts demanding more and more. By becoming addicted to sugar, you tend to eat it more often and in higher quantities—which leads to diseases that will put you in the grave early if you do not make the necessary changes. Sugar is every bit as dangerous as alcohol and tobacco—except it isn't being monitored and rarely taxed—and it is time that you learn to say no to this substance and move it out of your life.

My name is Alex and I am here to not only teach you why sugar is bad for you but also how to break your addiction from it to live a healthier and happier life. Every day I see the harm of sugar. Countless people are struggling to lose weight and get healthy by spending hours in the gym with little to no results. This is because their diet is sabotaging them. No matter how many hours you spend in the gym, if your diet isn't correct you will never lose those excess pounds. Since I was 16 years old I have been doing sports and working out. I noticed the subtle changes to my body—which were also improving the way I felt about myself—so I pushed myself to understand why this was happening. I studied nutrition to understand why it played a role in how a person can remain healthy and ended up with a degree in it. That isn't where I stopped; every day I am learning new nutritional knowledge that I aim to share with you in this book.

One of the first mistakes people make when they think about healthy food with no sugar is believing it has no taste and is boring. However, this book aims to show you that this is simply not true. It is just an excuse you are using to keep yourself in the cycle of poor eating. Eating healthily isn't just a choice; it is a necessity for someone to enjoy a long, healthy life.

I aim to show you that once you give up the addiction to sugar and other processed foods, you will be able to enjoy life more and live better. A healthy life can be achieved if you are willing to take the time to change habits and ignore negative influences in your life. The changes don't even need to be huge. It all starts with a decision. It only takes one small decision that could change your entire life by adding years to your lifespan and lowering your risk of early death. Just because sugar has a long history with the human race—and you —doesn't mean that it should have a place in your future. So, join me on this adventure to improve your confidence, drop those poor habits, and add extra years to your life by simply taking a closer look at what you eat and do.

1

THE UNKNOWN TRUTH ABOUT SUGAR

"A moment on the lips, a lifetime on the hips."

— UNKNOWN

I t is likely that you have read this saying before and realized that it was a warning about food that tastes great but could have nasty effects on your body. Everywhere you look, there are people making claims about certain food types not being good for the human body. This could be fat, carbohydrates, animal products, etc. and this has caused several diets to be designed to cut out these unwanted food types. Yet no one can agree on whether removing these sorts of foods is good for your health or not. However, the one thing that many people do agree upon is that processed foods and added sugars are the real problems to our modern diet—more than just one particular nutrient or food source.

Understanding what sugar is and what it is found in is a muddy affair because everything from fruit to bread contains some form of sugar. Not only that, but sugar comes in a variety of names—over 50 different names —which makes it more difficult to try and track your consumption of it. Several sugars are necessary for a healthy body while others are not that great for you. Sugar is a carbohydrate that comes in several forms which include monosaccharides (glucose or fructose), disaccharides (sucrose or lactose), oligosaccharides (raffinose or stachyose), fermentable polysaccharides (amylopectin or amylose), and non-fermentable polysaccharides (cellulose or pectin). Each has its own function and is used by the body in different ways. You cannot survive without consuming some of these types of sugars, as they give energy to complete daily tasks or provide a healthy gut biome.

But if sugar is necessary for a healthy body, then why is it demonized the way that it is? This is because people do not understand the difference between a naturally occurring sugar versus one that is refined or added to food due to human influence. Naturally occurring sugars come in the form of fruits, vegetables, milk, and grains—but these sugars do not stand alone. Foods like vegetables, grains, and fruit contain minerals, vitamins, fiber, and antioxidants alongside those sugars so there are several benefits to eating whole food. Fiber is particularly important as it helps to slow down the digestion of the sugars and prevents blood sugar spikes. Foods like dairy contain not only sugar (lactose) but also protein and calcium.

Meanwhile, processed and prepackaged goods are high in sodium and added sugar because these are the substances that help increase the shelf life of these products as well as making them tasty to us. Refined sugar can be found in just about everything you eat. You only need to turn the packaging around and look at the nutritional information to see if what you are eating contains sugar or not. And likely it does. To see how much total sugar you are consuming with your prepackaged meal only look under the carbohydrate section and you will note it. Added or refined sugar isn't just hidden in our food but we also willingly add it to our diets. Sodas and energy drinks are the worst of the offenders when it comes to people introducing sugar to their diet. Followed closely behind this are grain-based desserts, such as pie, and fruit juice. These are hardly the only problems. How much sugar do you add to your breakfast cereal or coffee in the morning? What about that powdered donut you had recently? Even a teaspoon of honey counts as added sugar, despite all the benefits you get from it.

Carbohydrates are one of the three essential macronutrients—the others being protein and fat—humans need to have a healthy life. These macronutrients make up certain portions of your diet. Portion control is important, and with sugar very few people can control the amount that they consume. Added sugar is not considered a necessary nutrient so it should be kept to a lower amount where possible, but this can be very difficult if you are not tracking the hidden sugars. It is easy enough to drop a teaspoon of sugar from your coffee but if you are still eating a powdered donut you are still introducing a high number of added or refined sugars and grains to your diet that can have a disastrous effect on your health and life in the long run.

ADDED SUGAR AND ITS EFFECTS

Americans are consuming a maximum of between 22 and 24 teaspoons (averaging about 17 teaspoons) of added sugar a day—either by adding it themselves or consuming hidden sugars through a variety of foods—which is about 350–380 calories every single day. These are calories that are not needed and generally go unnoticed for some time before a problem is noted. Excess calories, or energy, that aren't used by the body will be stored away for later use as fat. Increased storage of fat can lead to being overweight and then obesity. This excess eating of sugar can lead to problems such as cognitive decline, increased risk of cardiovascular disease (CVD), dyslipidemia (increased low-density lipoproteins and lower high-density lipoproteins), increased blood pressure, certain cancers, diabetes, and non-alcoholic fatty liver diseases. Consuming too much sugar affects almost all parts of your body.

Brain

When you eat sugar, it stimulates the pleasure center of your brain by causing a dopamine response. Dopamine is a neurotransmitter that influences your moods, your motivation, and gives you the feeling of pleasure. It makes you feel good. Unfortunately, it does not respond the same way when you eat whole food that contains natural sugars. This is why the pleasure center of your brain causes you to crave candy or sugary drinks over any kind of fruit. This sort of reaction by the brain forms an addictive response by the person experiencing it. This can lead to addictive behaviors if it is allowed to continue.

Your mood is also influenced by this interaction. You feel down, so you treat yourself to a candy bar. This mostly contains sugar which is quickly digested and causes a blood sugar spike almost immediately. Insulin is secreted to deal with high blood sugar, but sometimes too much is secreted to deal with very high blood sugar (sugar rush) and this can cause a high percentage of the sugar to be taken from your blood—leaving you with almost nothing. This is known as a sugar low or sugar crash. During a sugar crash, you may feel jittery or even experience anxiety. By continuing this vicious cycle of sugar highs and sugar crashes you can start to develop depression.

Even your neurotransmitters are influenced by sugar. If there is too much sugar in your body it causes the production of orexin to be lower and this causes you to feel tired and drowsy all the time.

Teeth

The bacteria that is the root cause of cavities love sugar and if you tend to indulge in too much they will breed out of control and cause damage to your teeth. Unless you are brushing your teeth after every single sugary treat, this bacteria will be multiplying with every added grain of sugar you consume.

Skin

Everyone wants to look younger than their true age; however, if you continue to eat excess sugar you will find that your skin starts to age prematurely. Collagen and elastin are the two types of protein fiber that keep your skin looking youthful and remaining firm. By consuming too much sugar you encourage your body to produce higher levels of advanced glycation end products (AGEs). The AGEs cause damage to the protein fibers of your skin, which can lead to the sagging of skin and the formation of wrinkles.

Joints

If you are someone who suffers from joint pain then it is best to avoid as much added sugar as possible. This is because sugar leads to inflammation which will affect areas that are already inflamed and painful.

Internal organs

Most of your important internal organs are affected by consuming vast quantities of sugar. A large number of foods that contain added sugars contain a type of sugar called fructose (fruit sugar) that is mostly digested by the liver. The liver breaks this type of sugar down and produces fat instead. This can result in non-alcoholic fatty liver disease (NAFLD) and non-alcoholic steato-hepatitis (NASH). If someone suffers from NAFLD then their liver has an unnatural buildup of fat around it, while if you are suffering from NASH you have a fatty liver that is not only inflamed but also scarred (steatosis). This scarring can start out small and only be a nuisance, but can lead to cirrhosis as it starts to cut off the blood supply to various parts of your liver.

By eating extra sugar you are forcing your body to produce more insulin than is needed and this can lead to your arteries becoming inflamed. Inflamed arteries are thicker and stiffer than normal ones. This causes your heart to have to work harder than it should. By placing more strain on this organ you increase the risk of heart attacks and strokes. People who consume between 17% and 21% of their total calories as sugar have a higher chance of developing a heart-related disease than those that consumed less sugar (Harvard Health Publishing, 2019).

Then there is the pancreas—the organ that produces the insulin. It is working tirelessly to try and control your blood sugar. If you are chronically forcing your pancreas to overwork, it will simply cease to function. Once a pancreas is no longer functioning the way it should, your blood sugar will no longer be correctly maintained and you will get type 2 diabetes and add more strain to your heart.

Not even your kidneys are safe! Blood sugar that is not maintained by insulin needs to be filtered from the blood and it is the kidneys that have this job. Unfortunately, the fine capillaries (blood vessels) that are found inside the kidneys get damaged by the high sugar content of the blood. Once the kidneys are no longer able to filter the sugar out it is noticed in the urine, which is one of the signs of kidney damage—which will lead to kidney failure if nothing is done about it.

Sexual Health

As the heart is affected, so is the circulatory system. If there is a problem with blood flow, then there can be no erections. Men who chronically eat too much sugar often find that they suffer from impotence or struggle to maintain healthy erections.

Hormonal Disturbances

Several hormones can be out of balance due to eating too much added sugar. The first is insulin. This hormone allows the liver, muscle, and fat cells to absorb excess sugar from your blood. If the body requires power to do anything, these cells release the stored energy for its use. If it isn't used, then it is turned into fat as a long-term storage method. However, if too much sugar is being pulled from the blood for storage this can cause the cells to become too full to take up any more sugar, which leads to insulin resistance. By becoming insulin resistant the cells that would normally take up the excess sugar from the blood no longer do and the blood sugar levels in the blood will not be managed and will start affecting the other organs in the body.

High levels of insulin have an effect on the growth hormone. Having lower growth hormone leads to a higher chance of abdominal obesity, a lower muscle mass, increased risk of type 2 diabetes, and even your libido will be affected.

Even the sex hormones are affected by sugar. Insulin resistance causes a drop in testosterone. In men, this can cause an increase in body weight, lowered muscle mass, and an increase in estrogen which leads to a lowered sex drive. Don't think you are off the hook, ladies! Although you produce smaller amounts of testosterone, you still produce and need it to ensure your sexual health is functioning the way it should. Women with lower than normal testosterone are prone to having higher body fat, lowered muscle mass, often feel scatterbrained, and have a lowered desire for sexual intercourse.

By continually eating high levels of sugar you can cause leptin resistance. The hormone leptin helps to regulate the feeling of being full. With leptin resistance, regardless of your body sending signals to your brain that you are full, your body fails to interpret the hormone correctly and therefore still thinks that you are hungry when you aren't. This can trigger you to overeat when you aren't hungry—leading to obesity.

High levels of insulin also cause the hormone cortisol (stress hormone) to increase and stay at high levels. When a person is constantly exposed to cortisol it leads to stress and causes feelings of anxiety and even depression.

Body Weight

The more insulin is required to store away excess sugar in the blood the more fat is being stored. This stored form of energy needs to be used or the body will simply continue to store away the sugar in as many cells as possible, which leads to an increase of weight over time.

Blood Pressure

Sugar's influence on blood pressure is numerous and some of this has been touched on already. One of the influences is that insulin resistance causes the mineral magnesium not to be as readily absorbed and causes it to be flushed from the body through urination. By having less magnesium in the body the blood vessels do not relax as readily and when they remain constricted it can raise your blood pressure.

Fructose causes an increase in uric acid that inhibits nitric oxide production. Nitric oxide is a vasodilator that is required by the body to maintain healthy blood pressure by opening up the blood vessels to allow more blood through. If the body doesn't produce enough nitric acid the vessels can remain constricted which will lead to an increase in blood pressure.

Even the AGEs, that are produced upon the consumption of sugar, can cause the stiffening of the blood vessels which can lead to diseases such as atherosclerosis. High levels of the hormones insulin and leptin also cause high blood pressure.

All of these diseases can lead to misery and increase the likelihood of an early grave, but not before spending an excessive amount of money trying to combat them. Yet how should it be fought against if it is in everything?

SHOULD SUGAR BE BANNED?

Even though several serious diseases are caused by sugar, not everyone is affected equally. Several of these diseases are not only influenced by sugar but also by the genetics of the person who is suffering from the disease. Some people are simply more predisposed to getting these diseases than others. Although people know that consuming large amounts of sugar isn't great for them it is difficult to know when to stop consuming it. This is because there has never been an upper limit determined for the consumption of sugar where it starts to cause problems in a person's health. However, it is known that humans do not need added sugar to survive as the body can get the energy it requires from the macronutrients consumed. As it stands today, people are eating up to four times the amount of added sugar than 40 odd years ago and the diseases associated with a poor diet are increasing exponentially every year to match this. Is it sugar? Is it processed food? What about refined grains? Likely it is a combination of all of these, with sugar leading the pack.

The American Heart Association recommends that a person consumes only 6 teaspoons (roughly 0.85 ounces) of sugar a day. A single 12-oz can of coke contains 39 g (9.75 teaspoons) of sugar, which is already over the recommended level of sugar consumption. Sodas are not the only problem. Sugar-sweetened drinks are one of the main reasons that people are consuming too many added sugar types. When a person drinks their calories instead of eating them they are left unsatisfied and may feel hungry again very soon. By not feeling satisfied, you will want to eat more; and since you have rewarded your brain with the sweet taste it wants more of that. This will rarely leave you wanting to reach for an apple to fill the hole in your belly.

Not only that, but excess fructose consumption, like high fructose corn syrup in sodas, can do the same damage to your liver as alcohol can do. At least with alcohol, you reach a point where you stop drinking because you overdose on it. Going back to the can of coke, consuming almost 10 teaspoons of sugar should cause the human body to vomit it up—yet it doesn't. This is because the phosphoric acid in the drink prevents you from doing so as it masks the intense sweetness. Yet people continue to drink it.

There have been several movements to lower the sugar content of sugary drinks—such as sugar tax or soda tax —yet that hasn't stopped the problems. Not all countries, let alone different states, are willing to do this. But why? Why is it so difficult to give up on using added sugars?

Toxic Food Environment

We all live in a toxic food environment. It doesn't matter if you are rich or poor, your need to buy food is driven by two main factors: addiction and convenience.

Sugar can be found in the majority of the food we eat and many industries are aware of this. Some of these are even aware of the dopamine responses and make use of it through neuromarketing. By creating a product that people develop a craving for, a client base will continue to pour money into the companies that produce these food types. Unfortunately, this just strengthens the addictive nature of people who in turn will struggle with giving up substances that are known to be bad for them. Unless this toxic food environment changes, it will be a difficult task to battle diseases such as type 2 diabetes and obesity.

As with other addictive substances, it isn't so easy to just drop sugar from your diet. This will result in consequences such as cravings, withdrawals, and then binging if your willpower is not strong enough. This just starts the vicious cycle all over again. The brain wants dopamine, and if a person only gets pleasure from eating food that is high in trans fats, sodium, and added sugars the cravings become a lot more difficult to combat. The brain will always want to go for foods that contain high calories as a survival mechanism and it doesn't always want to make the healthy choice. Apple or chocolate bar? Which one will give you more pleasure to eat?

Prepackaged foods are convenient for all. Who wants to come home every night to cook a full meal for a family when it is far more convenient to stop by a fast-food restaurant? You not only save time but you also save money. By saving time you think you can spend more time with your family. Saving money also causes your brain to feel less stressed because now you have extra money to spend on something else. However, are you really coming out as the winner of this situation when you are encouraging bad eating habits and becoming reliant on poor quality meals?

Small Changes

Consuming excess sugar is terrible for the human body. This is a known fact, yet people continue to eat sugar in quantities that cause several diseases and have life-changing consequences. Giving sugar up cold turkey is just as bad for you, but if you start small you can break the cycle of addiction. Gradual changes to your overall diet will help you to achieve this. Something as simple as adding one less teaspoon of sugar to your daily coffee or skipping that powdered donut once in a while is a good start. Meal prepping days in advance with home-cooked meals prevents you from going the convenient route to your closest fast food joint to get a meal. Dropping refined and prepackaged meals for whole foods is simple to do if you stick to a well-balanced shopping list. Switch your sugary drinks for water to quench your thirst. Then lastly, you do not have to do this alone. If you struggle with a food or sugar addiction, speak to your family physician to help you with a diet; or find someone else to talk to who can help you overcome this problem. Even the smallest change you make will help you in the long run for your health.

2

DECIDE TO IMPROVE YOUR HEALTH

W hy should you decide to improve your health? Many people are quick to point out all the negatives involved in a poor diet yet are slow to acknowledge the benefits of a healthy one. Instead of using the stick to scare yourself into a healthy diet, why not consider using the carrot approach?

WHY YOU SHOULD DECIDE TO BECOME HEALTHY

The first thing to realize is that a healthy lifestyle means different things to different people. Some people believe that to have a meaningful healthy life you need to jog five miles every single day, eat only organic foods, get enough sleep, and drink enough water.

Others may believe that a mile-long walk every day, spending time with the family creating a home-cooked meal, and getting to bed before 10 p.m. is a healthy lifestyle. The point is that both are correct for the kind of lifestyle that they want to lead. The definition of a healthy lifestyle is up to you to decide as you are the one who has to live it. As long as the lifestyle you lead doesn't cause you bodily harm or illness and aids in your health then it can be considered a healthy lifestyle.

The main reason that you want to have a healthy lifestyle is that a good diet and remaining active regularly prevents or lowers the risk of many problems, such as various heart diseases, type 2 diabetes, and cancer. By doing as little as 11 minutes of moderate to vigorous exercise every single day you can add years to your life in comparison to doing nothing and remaining in a sedentary lifestyle.

If you are improving your health you are saving money. By not becoming ill or combating serious or chronic diseases that can remain hidden—such as high blood pressure—you are saving thousands if not hundreds of thousands of dollars in doctors' bills. Yearly visits should still be done to keep an eye on biomarkers that can be an early warning sign of potential illnesses looming. Listen to the advice of your doctors to prevent possible diseases from developing. With a healthier lifestyle, your immune system is stronger which allows you to combat seasonal illnesses more easily than those who have weaker immune systems.

Leading a healthier lifestyle not only benefits you but also your environment. By choosing to eat fewer processed foods you are helping to lower greenhouse gas emissions, plastic waste, and a host of other environmentally devastating consequences. Instead of hopping in your car to go to the corner supermarket, you can use a bicycle or walk instead. By doing this for trips that are within a five-mile radius of your home you will be lowering your carbon footprint by producing fewer car emissions which means there will be less pollution in the air. Plus, you will be getting a workout.

You do not need to be a vegetarian or vegan to help the environment. By simply removing as little as a quarter pound of beef—or skipping a meat-based meal in favor of a plant-based meal—from the weekly meals, you are helping to lower the greenhouse gases produced by raising livestock at the scale that is needed to feed everyone in America.

Also, think of the example you will be setting for your children by adopting a healthier lifestyle. Children look to their parents' actions and shopping habits to form their opinions about food. By showing children which foods are better for their diet you can help combat one of the most serious problems that the United States is currently facing: childhood obesity. In 2018, a total of 14.4 million children under the age of 19 were obese (CDC, 2021). This was almost 20%—one in five—of the child population. This can be lowered in the future if the right food choices are made.

People who continue to consume poor diets end up in an early grave. Adopting a healthier diet, lifestyle, and doing regular exercise can add over a decade to your life. It pays to remain as healthy as possible. These are by no means the only benefits to be had when you choose to have a healthier lifestyle. Once you have decided to change your life for the better you will find that you become more focused, have more energy to do what you want, your sex life will improve, you will look and feel better which will lead to better self-esteem, you will be far happier, and your sleep will improve. All in all, making the change is a win-win situation for you.

HOW TO MAKE THE HEALTHY CHOICE

There is no one way to become healthy; there are many, which means you have many opportunities to make the change. The first thing you need to do is to decide that this is what you want to do. Not just decide but DECIDE. This acronym was coined by Kristina Guo

(2008) to help healthcare managers make decisions, but can easily be adapted to help you to decide to diminish the amount of added sugar you may be consuming in your diet.

Just thinking of making the change is an easy concept; however, the real challenge comes in making a solid plan that you can stick to and achieve. By having a plan in motion the correct changes can be made to help set you up for the success that you crave. Kristina Guo identifies six steps to help people build a solid decision-making model to help themselves:

- **D**: Define the problem.
- **E**: Establish criteria for the problem.
- **C**: Consider all possible alternatives.
- **I**: Identify the best possible alternatives.
- **D**: Develop, then implement, a plan of action.
- **E**: Evaluate and monitor the solution and provide feedback where needed.

Define the Problem

By knowing and understanding your problem it allows you to consider possible hurdles that may stand in your way of overcoming it. However, defining a problem can be rather tricky, and you have to be honest with yourself. For example, the problem isn't that you are overweight but rather that you are overweight because you have an addiction to sugar or food that is considered junk food. Once the problem has been identified, you need to consider why you want to change this. Continuing with the example, you want to lose weight because it will lead to a healthier life. The last question you will need to ask yourself is how the problem can be solved. If the problem is sugar addiction, you will need to give up or cut back on sugary goods.

Establishing Criteria

Setting up meaningful criteria is what is going to help you to get to your goal. There are three questions you will need to ask yourself before you can establish these criteria. The first is what do you want to achieve by giving up sugar? Perhaps you are doing this to lose weight, gain better health, or fit into an old favorite piece of clothing you haven't worn in a while.

The next question is what do you want to preserve about your current life? These could be criteria that you are unwilling to change because they are dear to you. Perhaps you have a sweet tooth that makes breaking the habit of eating sweet things too difficult or you may enjoy baking too much.

The last question is what problems do you want to avoid? An example of this would be not wanting to fall into the habit of binging on the incorrect foods because you are craving something sweet. Or being pressured into just trying a sugar-ladened treat by someone who refuses to respect or care about your health choices.

By having these criteria, you are pinpointing what you want and what you need to avoid. You want to achieve your goals without robbing yourself of things that you can't bear to part with. If a decision cannot satisfy all the criteria, it is not the type of decision you can stick to and you will need to change it or reevaluate your criteria. As with the example, giving up all sugars but not indulging a sweet tooth could cause a person to lose willpower and return to a poor diet. Whereas giving up added sugar still allows for sugar-free options or using fruit to handle the sweet tooth. Sugar in baking can be substituted for a variety of other sweetening agents that don't count as added sugar. All you need to do is look for possible alternatives.

Consider Alternatives

There will always be alternatives to help you reach your goals and you will need to consider them all before making a decision. To find these alternatives, you will have to do research, speak to professionals, or speak to people who have already achieved what you want to gain from this decision. A single alternative isn't enough—you will need several to help you make the right decision to get you closer to reaching your goal. Not all alternatives will be desirable or even obtainable and this is why you need several to choose from. Someone who has broken a leg, is healing from a wound, or is sick cannot combine rigorous exercise with diet to achieve weight loss, but they can adjust their calorie intake. They may take longer to reach their goal but they will still reach it.

Identify the Best Alternative

Out of all the alternatives you have researched, you may find there are several that best suit you and match the criteria you have set. Try to rank these alternatives against your criteria to see how they compare against each other and which will best benefit you with little to no undesirable effects. Don't be afraid to test each alternative to see which best suits your needs. When giving up added sugar, there are several ways to do this. You can use no added sugar or make the switch to some non-nutritional sweeteners that can either be artificial or natural. Alternatively, you can use dried fruits or fresh fruits to sweeten the baking or meals. There is no need to drop desserts from your meal plans when there are countless sugar-free varieties, including something as simple as a bowl of fruit salad with some fresh cream.

Develop and Implement Your Plan

By now you have chosen the alternative that best suits you and your needs. Now it is time to create and put a plan into motion. A decision without a plan is just going to fail before you can even get started. A plan gives a direction you want to go in; it helps you to anticipate possible changes and helps you to react correctly when something unexpected occurs. A sure way to stick to any kind of diet plan is to get meal plans that are designed for the purpose that best suits your goals. From these meal plans, you can decide what food in your home is going to aid you and what will hinder you. You can give away any food that will not suit your new lifestyle while putting together a shopping list to get what you need. Teach yourself to cook recipes that will help you with your goal and do lots of meal prepping. Having food prepared at home lowers the chance that you might make an excuse to stop at a fast-food restaurant to get food. The important thing to remember is that the changes will not be immediate. Therefore, give yourself at least 30 days before you decide whether it is working or not.

Evaluate and Monitor Your Plan

The only way to know whether your plan is working or not is to constantly monitor and evaluate it to see if there are any changes. These changes can be either good or bad. Just because you aren't losing weight doesn't mean that the plan isn't working. Look at other factors that could be changing, such as inches around the belly or being able to do more vigorous exercise. If these changes are occurring, then the plan is working and you should continue with what you are doing.

However, if nothing is changing—or you are feeling ill —you should go have your biomarkers checked. Biomarkers are indicators that measure certain biological states of the body. Biomarkers that are often checked are cholesterol, blood pressure, and blood sugar. If these markers are still high, you will need to review the contents of the food you are eating. Are they too high in additives, calories, or contain hidden sugars? Are you on medication that may need to be reevaluated now that you are on a diet to help manage symptoms of a disease? This is a good time to talk to your doctor or a registered dietician to help you with better meal plans. Or you may simply need more time on the diet.

To help you monitor your diet, start a journal in which you can document the food you eat, the calorie totals, biomarkers, and whatever else you wish. Use it to help you celebrate every little victory so that it is easier to remain happy with the decision that you made. It is vital that you remain honest with yourself or you will never be able to achieve your goals.

Sometimes, unexpected events can occur—even with the best-laid plans. You will need to be prepared to take steps to change your plan to overcome these events. Some artificial sweeteners cause upset stomachs or bloating, but that doesn't mean that you can't use them at all. Switch to something easier on your body and continue with your plan.

To help you evaluate your plan you will need to consider any possible problems that could occur while the plan is in motion—such as certain sweeteners causing adverse effects. Then consider what problems are more likely to occur than others. Will you have an aversion to a sweetener or will you feel like you do not have enough energy? What preventative steps can you take to avoid these problems or can they be avoided at all? If you are low on energy then likely you have not eaten the correct food or you failed to snack when your body needed it. This is an avoidable mistake that would not have happened if you had stuck to a meal plan. Reacting poorly to an artificial sweetener is a high possibility and is difficult to avoid unless one experiments. This is not an avoidable problem if you plan on using sweeteners.

Final Decision

No decision is foolproof, so you may find that you need to tweak your plan as you go along with this journey. As long as you stick to the criteria that you determined, then your plan can simply evolve as you need it to.

STEPS TO TAKE TO BECOME HEALTHY

You have made your decision. You have a plan ready to go. But is that all you should do? By establishing that you have a problem, you can sit down and work on a goal that you want to achieve by the end of your plan. Do not limit yourself to a single goal but rather have the main goal—something that will be achievable in the long run—and several goals that are more easily achievable in the short term. Know how you want to measure your successes. Don't just stick to weighing yourself, as this can cause you to feel depressed if you do not see the scale moving. Consider using measurements such as biomarkers or even inches so that you can see some sort of improvement even though the scale says that there is none.

Once your goals are set you need to realize that this isn't something that is going to just occur overnight. You need to be willing to put the time and effort into it. Meal prepping is vital to a diet but can take a chunk of your time until you know what you are doing. However, it will be worth it when your health starts to improve.

Your diet will need a complete revamp but this doesn't mean that it will cost you an arm and a leg. Incorporate more fruits and vegetables into your diet. The more variety and colors you can get the better for your health. Create colorful salads from different kinds of fruits and vegetables to get a wider range of benefits as well as increasing the number that you eat. Ensure that you are only using whole fruits and vegetables, as these contain the most benefits for you. An apple is far better for you than a glass of apple juice.

Start out small. Add fruit to your breakfast to give you the sweetness you may be craving. Berries in oats is a refreshing breakfast that is packed with energy and antioxidants. Meals that don't have a type of fruit should have at least one type of vegetable. If you are already eating a vegetable with a meal add a different kind or two to bring more fiber and color to your diet.

Remove any refined grains, and goods made with them, from your home. Swap them out for whole grains so that you don't feel that you are missing something in your diet. Trade that white bread for multigrain bread while those sugary cereals can easily be replaced with some oats cooked with cinnamon to give you a tasty and filling breakfast.

Unless you are partaking in any fasting practices, always eat breakfast. It is called breakfast for a reason. You have been sleeping for hours and it is time for you to break that fast by eating something wholesome that will last you to your next meal.

Cook from home. Not only will this help you in your meal preparation but since you are making it you know exactly what is going into the meal and can avoid using items that contain added sugar. You can also practice portion control at home as it is easy to store away food that has not been eaten. Too often we feel that we must clean our plates while at a restaurant—when it is not needed—and this leads to overeating. By portion controlling what you eat, you limit the number of calories you are consuming. Fewer calories eaten leads to less excess weight. When cooking, opt to always cook with healthy fats such as avocado and olive oil while limiting fats like butter and avoiding all artificial trans fats, such as margarine.

Always have healthy snacks on hand! Snacks are vital as they prevent your blood sugar from dipping too low while you wait for the main meal. As long as the snacks are high in fiber, full of taste, and contain no added sugar or additives then they can be eaten to give you the energy you need to wait till your next meal. What is in these snacks needs to be monitored as too many can lead to consuming more calories than what you may wish. Freshly chopped vegetables with homemade hummus is a great snack. Alternatively, have some fruit salad with some yogurt. If those don't tickle your fancy then try some of the recipes in Chapter 4 to help you overcome your sweet tooth.

You need to increase your activity level. A short walk daily is far better than doing absolutely nothing. Exercise strengthens your muscles, helps with balance, and improves cardio health. Start small by trying to do 10 minutes of exercise every day and then build it up to the majority of your week having 30-minute sessions. Exercise doesn't mean that you have to run—unless you want to—you can walk, ride a bicycle, swim, or even try yoga. Do what best suits your lifestyle needs.

When you want to quench your thirst, stop reaching for the soda or even diet soda. Only water should be used to quench your thirst, while other drinks should only be had for enjoyment or relaxation. Avoid adding sugar to your coffee or tea or drinking sugar-laden drinks.

Get enough sleep and rest. Observe healthy bedtime hygiene by avoiding too much screen time before bed, monitoring the temperature and light in your bedroom, and going to bed at a reasonable time to get enough rest that best suits your needs. Many people like to say eight hours is enough, but this isn't true for everyone. Exercise is needed for a healthy life but you also need to know when to take a break and allow your body the rest it needs to recover from training sessions.

Try to manage your stress levels. This is something that many people struggle with daily but you must do it. Your body isn't designed to handle high levels of cortisol for extended periods as this can lead to similar problems that are seen in people that eat excess amounts of added sugar. Stress can be managed through exercise—through the release of endorphins—relaxing with friends, journaling, and taking up meditation. However, if you cannot manage your stress levels by yourself seek professional help. A therapist will be able to give you the necessary techniques to help you manage your stress successfully.

You do not need to do this alone. Humans are a gregarious species which means that most people like to have some kind of human interaction from time to time. Feelings of isolation can lead to depression and loneliness. Something as simple as a chat with a neighbor over the fence, organizing a Skype or Zoom call with friends, or having a friendly interaction with a cashier is enough to lower the feeling of being alone. And remember to reach out to your friends who may also need this kind of interaction.

DROPPING BAD HABITS

Giving up bad habits can be a very challenging thing to do, and for some people, it can be just about impossible. This just highlights that alternatives are needed to make your plan work for you. Look for possible alternatives to a poor habit and replace it or lower the frequency of which you do this poor habit. And if you falter, remember the most important thing; you are human and sometimes you make mistakes. Be kind to yourself and remember that hurtful words damage you far more than a poor habit ever could. It was a mistake; mistakes can be fixed. Pick yourself up and try again. A single mistake shouldn't have to define you forever. This is a journey, so expect a few stubbed toes now and again. It is only a failure if you give up, not if you continue forward. It will get easier until you no longer do or even think about a poor habit. It just takes some time.

3

FIRST STEPS TO SAYING NO

Addiction is an event that doesn't happen overnight. It is something that starts out small that eventually grows into something you can no longer live without or are able to control. This may even be ruining your life either physically, mentally, or emotionally. A person can become addicted to many different kinds of things which are not limited to illegal substances, such as drugs, but also legal drugs, such as alcohol or over-the-counter medications—yet these are hardly the only examples. These are just the examples that people are willing to get help for with enough convincing.

Although sugar isn't seen as damaging as many other legal or illegal substances, it still causes your brain to go through the same patterns of withdrawal and cravings.

There are some people that state sugar is as addictive as heroin or cocaine. And, as with all types of addictions, sometimes you are capable of handling the situation by yourself but other times you will need a little help. The first thing you need to do is admit to yourself that you have a problem and then get the help you may need to heal your life.

ARE YOU ADDICTED?

There is a feeling of guilt associated with being an addict and many people are not willing to see that their actions are proof of this. There are several signs of an addiction—which outsiders can see easier than you can —that you will need to notice before you acknowledge that there is a problem. Many people tend to deny that they have a problem and will even go out of their way to deny that their habit is the cause of the problems in their life. Being able to admit that you have a problem is the first sign of wanting something better for yourself.

How to Tell That You Are Addicted

You are constantly craving all manner of sweet carbohydrates and then feel guilty when you overindulge in your favorite treat. You continue to eat these sweet treats despite not being hungry. If someone points out this poor eating habit to you, you feel that you must immediately defend your eating habits and even justify why you eat this way. After an indulging session, you are often left feeling sluggish and extremely moody. The very thought of having to give up sugar makes you break out in a cold sweat.

Does this sound like you? If so, then you are likely addicted to sugar. By consuming high levels of sugar constantly, you not only fuel the habit but you are cementing the addictive behavior that will prevent you from being able to tackle the growing problem.

Dealing with the Physical Aspects

The food you eat can either fuel addiction or help you break away from it. Everything you consume contains some form of sugar. Using a carbohydrate calculator— such as Carb Manager—can aid you in determining the number of carbs and sugars you eat. With the help of these kinds of apps, you should be able to police your eating habits a little better.

It isn't just added sugars that you need to be concerned about when you suspect that you have a sugar addiction. Your choice of carbohydrates can also influence how much sugar is made available to your body. Foods that contain simple carbohydrates are digested quickly and give a lot of sugar that spikes your insulin quickly, while complex carbohydrates take longer to digest and release sugar slower throughout the day. However, in severe cases of sugar addiction, when you cannot control your eating habits, you may need to switch to a diet that heavily controls the number of carbohydrates that you eat. These carb-conscious diets include the keto, Paleo, and Atkins diets.

Even if you are monitoring your sugar levels carefully, you are fighting a battle with your brain which is yearning for a quick dose of dopamine to get it through the day. When the brain doesn't get this, it will start craving any and all kinds of sugary treats. When it is not fed what it demands, it will go into withdrawal which can be a painful process, as the pleasure center of the brain is close to where it interprets pain. To relieve this pain you feel compelled to just have a tiny amount of sugar. By doing this, you will only cause the cycle to restart and all your hard work will be for nothing.

Why do we crave sugar so much? It goes back to childhood experiences that you have been taught. Humans love to celebrate all kinds of achievements and this is usually accompanied by some kind of sugary treat. When it is someone's birthday you consume all sorts of baked goods, candies, and sugary drinks. When a child cries adults tend to give them some candy to calm down. When adults have a bad day they like to relax with some kind of a drink that is usually high in carbs. This behavior is reinforced time and time again, so it is no wonder that humans turn to sugar as their first line of defense when anything goes right or wrong.

A sure way to break away from this sort of behavior is to completely remove the temptation and avoid situations like those mentioned above. However, this isn't always possible as there may be people in your life that simply won't respect your wishes or they themselves continue to eat high levels of sugars and carbohydrates which can lead to you being tempted. You may even be forced to avoid places where it has been easy to indulge your habit in the past.

A sure way to deal with sugars in your diet is to replace them with something else. One of the diets that many people turn to is the keto diet, not only because it forces you to eat fewer sugars but to replace them with good quality, healthy fats. A single gram of fat gives you nine calories worth of energy while a gram of carbohydrates and protein each only gives you four grams. By keeping your fat intake high, your protein moderate, and carbohydrates to a minimum (usually by consuming fruits and vegetables that are high in fiber) you stand a good chance of conquering your physical need for sugar.

To aid in ridding yourself of the sugar cravings, you will need to remove all obvious sources of added sugar such as granulated sugars, syrups, etc. After this, you will need to get rid of processed foods that contain high levels of fructose corn syrup or other added sugars. Finally, you will need to give up simple carbohydrates in favor of complex carbohydrates. The keto diet not only cuts out sugars but also a large number of carbohydrates. There are many different kinds of keto diets that you can try so you are sure to find one that best suits you.

The most commonly followed of the keto diets is the standard keto diet (SKD). This diet allows for 70–80% of your diet to consist of fat, 15–20% protein, and 5–10% carbohydrates. By not providing the body with carbohydrates, it can no longer use sugar as a form of energy. Your body is forced to switch from glycolysis to ketosis—which is the burning of ketones, a product of fat digestion—for energy, as you are providing a different macronutrient as a form of energy. There is more stored energy inside a single fat molecule than there is in glucose so your body can make the switch in just a few days. By entering ketosis your body is using fat to power it, and not just from the types of fat that you eat but also from the fat stored in your body. This diet has been known to help with weight loss, easing or reversing type 2 diabetes (as it helps with controlling your glucose level and insulin sensitivity), and helping with childhood epilepsy. Although this diet concentrates heavily on the consumption of fat it shouldn't just be any fat. Healthy fats from both animal and plant sources are encouraged while artificial fats and all processed foods are discouraged. This diet can also help with curbing hunger, as by consuming higher levels of fat you become more sated and the feeling of fullness lasts longer. This prevents overeating and unnecessary excess snacking. It is very important to keep your carbohydrate intake to 10% as consuming more will prolong the time it takes to get into ketosis. Similarly, the consumption of protein needs to remain at a moderate 20% or the body will convert it to glucose through gluconeogenesis (conversion of non-carbohydrate molecules to glucose.) There are bodily functions that still require carbohydrates to function and the body will create them if it is needed.

However, be warned that when starting a keto diet you will go through a phase known as keto flu. Your body is used to using glucose as a source of energy and when you take that away from it you will go through the same withdrawals as you would with when you stop using sugar. Some of the symptoms may include nothing more than headaches and cravings, while it can be more severe with instances of nausea, stomach issues, and vomiting. That is the kind of hold that carbohydrates have on your life. This is not an easy diet to stick to and if you are suffering from any form of kidney disease it is suggested that you do not try this diet. It can also be particularly difficult for people who suffer from obsessive-compulsive disorder (OCD) as micromanaging their diet can lead to eating disorders. This diet can also be difficult for people who love to train in the gym as they do not have their stored glucose to help them through their training sessions.

However, there are several variations to the keto diet that help those that want to work out. There is the cyclical keto diet (CKD), which allows for five days of a strict keto diet and then two days where you can reintroduce more carbohydrates to your diet. You want to be using complex carbohydrates as you want the carbohydrates to digest slowly. The days that you are eating carbohydrates are called re-feed days and it is how you replenish your glucose stores in your muscles. Unfortunately, this will kick you out of ketosis. However, if you practice this for a long time, returning to ketosis becomes easier.

Then there is the targeted keto diet (TKD) which tries to preserve the ketosis state of your body. By consuming a small meal of simple carbohydrates before a training session—about 45 minutes before your session—your body will use the glucose produced to fuel itself. The training session should be strenuous enough to burn through all the glucose while not allowing any to be stored in the muscles for later use. Whichever diet you decide to choose, be sure to monitor how much sugar you consume and if you are in ketosis. This can be done by testing ketones found in the blood, urine, or breath.

If you are interested in trying the keto diet it gets a little more difficult. It isn't just about cutting out the known carbs such as rice or potatoes. You will also need to take a closer look at what fruit and vegetables you want to eat. You will need to remove a large number of fruits and vegetables that contain more than 10 g of net carbs (digestible carbohydrates) per 100 g. Those that follow this type of diet that wish to be more controlling of their carbohydrate intake may even consider dropping the allowance of net carbs to 5 g of net carb per 100g of fruit or vegetable consumed. Due to the low percentage of carbohydrates allowed on the keto diet, you should always go for fruits and vegetables that have high fiber contents to help with any possible digestive concerns.

Strict dietary control is only one way you can manage the physical aspects of addiction. You will need to learn how to recognize, avoid, or deal with triggers that cause you to crave sugar. When unavoidable cravings strike, look for ways to distract yourself until the feeling disappears. Exercise or hobbies are great distractions. Reach out and talk with people you trust about how the cravings make you feel and the struggles you are going through. They may even have advice for you on how to deal with what you are going through. Remind yourself why giving in to a craving is bad for you. Alternatively, you can attempt to ride out the craving through urge surfing. By mindfully focusing on the urge and why it is there you will learn to overcome it.

Overcoming addiction is going to take a lot of time, motivation, and the support of those around you. You may need to constantly remind yourself why you are going through this, especially when it starts to get difficult. This is where you will need to be strong and reach out to those that can support you. There is no shame in asking for help. Be sure to stick to any goals that you want to achieve as these will be the beacons to show that you are succeeding. Is this your first time trying to give up sugar? If not, use past failed attempts to see what helped or hindered your previous attempt. Consider what is stopping you from dropping this poor habit and see if it is a real reason or a pathetic excuse. Lastly, consider the pros and cons of kicking a habit that is slowly killing you. There will be more pros than cons.

However, sometimes the addiction is more than just a physical occurrence. Sometimes it is nothing more than a symptom of a larger problem that you are burying under a mountain of snacks because you simply do not want to deal with it. There are times that nothing seems to be working—you have given up sugar for some time but the cravings just will not go away—and now the cravings are interfering with your life. This is when you need to consider that your addiction may no longer be physical but rather emotional.

Dealing with the Emotional Aspect

The brain demanding a dopamine boost is a physical aspect, but when this has been addressed by other means and the cravings seem to continue, then likely you have an emotional bond with sugar. By only concentrating on the physical aspect of addiction, the emotional aspect will continue to fester and cause problems even though you haven't eaten sugar in some time.

Emotional addiction has its own signs—though some signs are similar to physical addiction—that allow you to recognize it for what it is. The first sign is that even after a sugar detox you can't wait to eat some sugar. You feel anxious about not being able to eat sugar. It seems to be the only thing that keeps you calm during times of stress, or when you feel excited or sad. You also tend to associate the feeling of safety and comfort with consuming sugar.

Similar to the physical addiction, the emotional bond didn't form overnight. Something as simple as when you were a child and you scraped a knee may have started it. Your parents likely placated you with a candy bar while they tended to your wound. This caused an association with pain being diminished through the eating of sugar. Or perhaps one day you were feeling sad and your parents took you out for ice cream. Because of this, the feeling of banishing sadness is now associated with a sugary treat. Similarly, parents try to soothe a child who has gone through trauma with gifts or treats. When this happens often enough it gets ingrained in our subconscious as being okay and then you continue that behavior when you are an adult.

This can also give rise to emotional eating. As seen with celebrating events and achievements, sugary food can be seen as a reward system. As much as people love this reward system, it is actually a poor coping mechanism that can cause ingrained behaviors that can be difficult to break people of. Emotional hunger cannot be sated by any kind of food which acts as a temporary fill to a hole that needs emotional support. By feeding an emotional hunger you are contributing to the emotional eating cycle. Something upsets you, which triggers the feeling of wanting to eat something. You eat until you no longer feel upset, inevitably causing you to overeat. By overeating, you start to feel guilty which triggers a fresh turning of this vicious cycle.

Because you have been taught to eat your feelings away you don't seek alternatives to help you with your emotional issues. Why would you? Your history shows that food numbs the pain or makes you feel better. This way of dealing with emotional problems is quicker, easier, and more satisfying than dealing with a problem head-on and finding a real solution.

Before you can even begin to deal with the emotional bond you may have with sugar you need to deal with the emotional eating first. Many people struggle to realize the difference between true hunger and emotional hunger, leading them to eat whenever they feel a pang of hunger without considering if they really are hungry or not. Physical hunger—where you truly are hungry—develops over several hours and can be satisfied by any kind of meal. The hunger pangs originate from the belly and when you are eating there is no guilt involved as you need the nutrients in the food to survive and have a healthy life. True hunger stops once you are full and is managed through mindfully eating your food.

Emotional hunger suddenly occurs and is normally triggered by something happening to you. You will have cravings for something specific and nothing else will do except that specific type of food. There are no true hunger pangs, as it is all in your head. Once you have finished eating what your cravings have told you to eat you find yourself feeling ashamed and guilty for eating it. You may feel that it was nothing more than empty calories and eating something else would have been far better for you. When eating in this state you will rarely concentrate on what you are eating and will mindlessly graze until you literally feel sick from eating so much.

To treat emotional eating you will need to figure out what your triggers are and how you can deal with them. These triggers can include boredom or feeling empty, poor habits learned from childhood, stress, and even social influences. Perhaps you feel obligated to clean your plate even when there is too much food on it for you. This is something that does lead to overeating.

Find ways to avoid these emotional traps by looking for alternative ways to deal with them. If you are feeling lonely or depressed then reach out to people around you. When feeling anxious, do something to distract you from the feeling. Exercising with some music is a great way to distract yourself. Feeling exhausted? Don't reach for the hot chocolate. Make a cup of tea, or relax in a bath with some bubbles, or pick up a good book. No one should ever suffer from boredom. Go out and discover a new hobby, go exploring—practically anything else except eating. Finding alternative ways to deal with your triggers doesn't mean that you are denying the feelings associated with the cravings you feel. Cravings are normal and so are the feelings associated with them. By accepting both of them you are well on your way to healing.

When you feel a craving hit you take a moment to distract yourself from the feeling and think about the emotions that are playing a role at that very moment. What emotion are you currently feeling? What is the best way to deal with this emotion? Spoiler alert: It isn't food.

The emotional bond you have with sugar can't simply be broken but requires a healthier bond to replace it. Only then can you fully heal from addiction. These replacement bonds should include a healthy relationship with yourself and those around you. This should be what you turn to when things don't work out in your life. Cravings for things you shouldn't eat may always be at the back of your mind but if you treat them kindly instead of with fear or guilt they will become easier to deal with as you learn to manage them better while on this journey. By combating the feelings of anxiety and guilt associated with cravings they become easier to accept as part of your life and therefore break the emotional bond they hold over you.

To heal from this bond you need to make a note of what sugar does to you. Are there destructive patterns you tend to follow when consuming sugar? Can you control your consumption? This will help you judge what kind of choices you will need to make when giving up these sweet goods. Don't forget to do self-care. Giving an addiction up is hard work. You need to not only treat your body well but also your mind. Encourage yourself with kind words, cook well-balanced meals, take time out of the day for just you, enjoy good sleep, and drink plenty of water. Acknowledge when you have slip-ups on this journey. Don't hide them. Don't curse at this failure. Encourage yourself to try again, documenting where you went wrong and finding alternatives to help you overcome this bump in the road. If you have a journal, document your feelings and acknowledge them without guilt-tripping yourself. And when the addiction feels bigger than you, seek professional help. You are not alone in this. An addiction is an addiction, no matter what you are addicted to and many professionals can help you.

Relapses

They are going to happen. There is no way around it. Maybe you will be lucky and you find the best alternatives using the DECIDE method and you never relapse. Or maybe you stumble and fall on your very first day. You need to realize that a relapse is not a failure. Yes, there are health implications involved if you do not stop eating sugar in excess, but relapse is not going to result in the failure of this journey. A relapse is a chance to reflect on what went wrong—was it emotional, physical, or a particular person. Write down everything so that you know what to look out for in the future when you try again. The only way that a relapse turns into a failure is when you give up completely. Try again; you have it in you.

HOW TO SAY NO TO SUGAR

You will need to use a combination of both willpower and emotional strength to get through turning away from sugar. You may stumble a few times, but in the end, you will get to the goal that you want to achieve. Several healthy alternatives were already discussed in Chapter 2.

Find out why you are turning to sugar as your first food choice when you are feeling stressed out. There is likely an underlying situation you will need to deal with before you can move forward with successfully saying no to sugar.

When you are exhausted or staying up very late, your body is going to crave sugar as a form of quick energy to keep you going or to keep you awake. By getting adequate levels of sleep you can avoid not only consuming sugar but also excess calories you do not need.

Consider the reason for going on this journey in the first place. Are you doing it out of fear or obligation? No one responds well to those limitations. Perhaps consider changing the way you view the situation and change this experience into a more positive one. This will help you learn to love yourself again and therefore make the journey an easier one with a lot less guilt associated with it.

Don't equate the taste of sugar for food tasting good. There are many ways to make food tasty without having to resort to any form of added sugar. Teach yourself to cook and prepare food with different kinds of spices. Spices like cardamom, cloves, and cinnamon have long been used by people all over the world to bring out the sweetness of dishes.

If there are people in your life that keep trying to get you to eat what you are trying to give up then it is perhaps time to reevaluate your relationship with them. This is going to be a difficult enough journey without having someone sabotaging your goals. Surround yourself with people who are going to support you and not keep you in a state where your health is constantly deteriorating.

Be careful when just replacing your usual amount of sugar with a similar amount of alternative sweetener. Some of them are far sweeter than regular sugar and therefore need to be used in smaller amounts than sugar. There is a wide range of products that you can use—such as sugar alcohols or novel sweeteners—you will need to see which best suits your needs. Artificial sweeteners, however, can be a double-edged sword. This is because they still provide that sweet taste and this can trigger cravings that are difficult to manage. Despite this, these sugar alternatives are an excellent way to help most people give up added sugar with a few benefits to your health. The FDA considers most modern-day sweeteners to be generally recognized as safe (GRAS). So much so that even pregnant women can use them.

And lastly, practice the word no. When someone asks you if you want sugar in your coffee, say no. When you are offered a slice of cake or dessert, say no. You are invited to a birthday party where you know there will be sweet treats to tempt you. Say yes. Being on a journey where you are limiting your intake of sugar shouldn't prevent you from going to social events. Take your own sugar-free or alternative foods with you after you explain to your host why you are doing this. True friends will be accepting of a change that means your health improves and you will be around longer to celebrate more birthdays.

4

REPLACING SUGAR

As an addictive substance, it can be exceedingly difficult to give sugar up cold-turkey. It isn't just the physical addiction that you will need to combat but also the emotional side. If you think you will struggle with giving up sugar, look to alternatives to help you along your journey.

SWEETENERS

The term sweeteners is used for anything that sweetens what you are consuming. There are many types that you can use to help you get over your addiction. Some are better than others in not only taste but also the number of calories they have. Many sweeteners are considered safe for human consumption but there are little to no—or even outdated—studies that look at the long-term risks of consuming such products. Some may even need more human studies to give us the full picture behind each one. Consuming in moderation is the safest bet with all of these products.

Natural Sweeteners

Natural sweeteners can be divided into two groups. Those that are only slightly better than regular sugar and those that make perfect alternatives to using sugar that contain little to no sugar. Of the best natural sweeteners, there is a plant-based product called stevia. This sweetener is extracted from the leaves of the plant *Stevia rebaudiana* and is considered to be significantly sweeter than regular sugar. It contains no calories and tastes exactly like sugar with no strange aftertaste. Stevioside—a compound found in stevia—is known to lower blood sugar—which in turn lowers insulin responses—as well as helping to reduce blood sugar.

A sweetener can also be extracted from the monk fruit (Luo Han Guo) that yields no calories that isn't quite as sweet as stevia but is still considerably sweeter than regular sugar. Although the fruit contains both fructose and glucose it isn't these sugars that give the sweetener its sweetness. During the process of creating this product, the compound mogroside is separated from the juice of the fruit while the fructose and glucose remain behind. These mogrosides are not only sweet but also provide anti-inflammatory properties and antioxidants. This product doesn't influence insulin or blood sugar levels.

Yacón syrup is from the plant *Smallanthus sonchifolius* and has an appearance similar to that of molasses. Although this is a syrup—which should normally be avoided—it contains 50% fructooligosaccharides that cannot be digested by the body. This is a type of carbohydrate that has many benefits including having a reduced glycemic index (GI), helps manage body weight, and lowers the risk of colon cancer. It also assists in producing a healthy gut biome which in turn lowers the risk of diabetes and obesity. Per gram of this syrup, you will get 1.3 calories.

There are several other natural sweeteners that you can use if you want to slowly break away from regular sugar. However, these sweeteners are still very high in sugar and are only slightly better than regular sugar.

Coconut sugar has a lower GI than regular sugar and contains a soluble fiber called inulin. This fiber helps to digest the sugar more slowly, helps to feed the various gut microbes (good bacteria, viruses, and fungi), and can help you feel fuller for longer. However, this type of natural sugar is still very high in fructose.

Honey is one of the natural sweeteners that many people like to turn to due to the benefits it offers. It is high in antioxidants from flavonoids and phenolic acids which are known to help with the prevention of inflammation, diabetes, cancers, and even heart disease. However, this contains a high concentration of fructose.

If you are not a fan of honey perhaps you would prefer maple syrup? This syrup contains even more antioxidants than honey as well as minerals such as potassium, calcium, manganese, and zinc. Several test tube and rodent studies have shown that there are benefits to consuming maple syrup. This includes lowering the plasma glucose concentrations as well as helping with type 1 diabetes. However, the GI is only slightly smaller than that of sugar and it will still cause a blood sugar spike. There are also no human studies to date.

If you have to choose a natural sweetener, the lesser of all the natural sugar evils is molasses. This product has a few antioxidants but is full of minerals such as iron, potassium, and calcium which go a long way in strengthening your bones and heart.

Sugar Alcohols

There are two sugar alcohols that you can use as sweeteners. The first is erythritol. Of the two sugar alcohols, this one has the lowest number of calories per gram at only 0.24. This is only 6% of the calories that a gram of sugar contains. It also tastes similar to sugar and many people use this to make the switch. The human body lacks the necessary enzymes in which to completely digest erythritol, because of this the sweetener is absorbed and excreted virtually unchanged. This prevents your blood sugar and insulin from being impacted by it. It also doesn't affect total cholesterol or triglycerides. This is a very safe sweetener to use but can tend to be a little expensive due to the processing costs of making it.

The second sugar alcohol is xylitol. The taste is almost like sugar but tends to have a cooling aftertaste—similar to mint—and contains 2.4 calories per gram. Although higher in calories this sweetener doesn't contain fructose—the sugar that causes most of the health problems—and so doesn't cause a spike in blood sugar or insulin response. This sweetener needs to be used in moderation as at high dosages many people tend to experience digestive issues. This sweetener is toxic to dogs so if you have a furry friend at home be sure that they cannot get to it or use something else.

Artificial Sweeteners

Sometimes you won't find natural sweeteners to be at your disposal; especially at a coffee house when you are looking for something to sweeten your drink. You may need to turn to some artificial sweeteners to help you with this. There are several products that you can use. One of the most frequently used—especially in sugar-free drinks—is sucralose. This sweetener is exponentially more sweet than sugar and you should only ever use a tiny amount when using it. It cannot be metabolized by the body and therefore provides zero calories and makes it perfect for the keto diet. It doesn't leave a bitter aftertaste but it cannot be used for cooking or baking. Because of its intensely sweet taste, it is often spliced with sweeteners before being marketed. One of the products that contain sucralose is Splenda. Although sucralose has zero calories Splenda does, as it also contains maltodextrin and dextrose—two types of carbs—and each pack consumed will result in three calories being consumed.

Saccharin—which has a metallic aftertaste—is another artificial sweetener that is found in Sweet 'N Low in combination with dextrose. Another sweetener that is combined with dextrose is aspartame—which is the least sweet of the artificial sweeteners—and is known under the name Equal. Aspartame has been known to cause several allergic reactions that range from severely swollen lips and even anaphylaxis so be wary when using products that contain it.

Avoid at All Costs

Some products are labeled as healthy alternatives to added sugar but they may contain more sugar than regular sugar so it is important to check your nutritional labels before purchasing anything. One such product is agave syrup. This product comes from the same plant that is used to make tequila. Unfortunately, the syrup is 85% fructose which is higher than what regular sugar has.

High fructose corn syrup is another product you need to avoid at all costs. Although it is rare to find it as a product on its own, it is often found in all manner of processed food. To see which products may contain it, look at the nutritional information list at the back of all foods.

Maltodextrin is a highly processed sweetener that is literally no different from regular sugar. If a package of something says sugar-free but it contains maltodextrin then know you are still consuming the same amount of calories of sugar, just under a different name.

FRUIT USED AS SWEETENERS

Perhaps you want other possible alternatives to your sugar needs when it comes to recipes that contain sugar. You already turn to fruit as a natural sugar replacer for snacks so why not give fruit a try in cooking? Before you start to substitute the below fruit for sugar, you need to realize why sugar is used in a recipe —especially in baking. Sugar isn't just there for the sweetness; it is there to do several vital jobs. Sugar goes through a chemical change with the other ingredients that allow it to create a structure and in some recipes provide a browning effect. Not all recipes will come out the same way if you simply just replace sugar. Look to use recipes that have added texture in them—like the addition of oats—as these will be the recipes that will likely not be as affected by having the sugar switched out.

If you go ahead with substituting the added sugar you may need to play around with the recipe as the addition of different kinds of fruit will have an influence on the liquid content of the recipe. For example; a cup of unsweetened applesauce—or a cup and a half depending on your needs—can replace a cup of sugar, but you will need to use between ¼–⅓ cup less liquid such as milk or water. Applesauce also makes for a great egg replacement if you are a vegan.

Figs are another great fruit that you can use to replace sugar. This fruit is high in fiber, potassium, iron, and calcium which is perfect for strengthening your bones, digestive system, and helps you to have healthy blood. Take eight ounces of fresh figs with ¼–⅓ cup of water and add it to a food processor, then blend until you have a smooth mixture. This mixture can be substituted on a 1:1 ratio with sugar. You can also use dry figs for this but you will need to soak them before pureeing them. Remember that dried fruit contains more sugar than fresh fruit. Compensate appropriately. This puree also makes wonderful sugar-free jams and jellies. With a little more water added you can create a liquid fruit syrup that you can add to your preferred drinks to help sweeten them.

Overripe bananas can now help you replace sugar instead of rotting away or waiting to be made into banana bread. This fruit is an excellent source of fiber and potassium which will help you control your blood pressure naturally. A cup of overripe, mashed banana with just enough water to turn it into a puree is enough to replace a cup of sugar. You may find that you will need to lower the liquid part of the recipe by two to three tablespoons. Bananas are also good as egg replacements.

Another great fruit that is often used to replace sugar is dates. This fruit is high in calcium, iron, phosphorus, copper, manganese, and fiber. They are excellent for the blood, stomach, and bones. All you need is a cup of pitted dates with ½–1 cup of hot water blended until it becomes a paste before replacing a cup of sugar. If you are using date sugar you will need ⅔ of a cup to replace a cup of sugar.

These are by no means the only fruits that you can use to help with switching out sugar. Citrus fruit like the Meyer lemon is very sweet and you can add some of its juice to your cooking instead of sugar. Grapefruit—the red ones tend to be nice and sweet—and lime can be added to drinks to give them a refreshing zing that is sure to squash your need for sugar.

Raisins and cranberries—dried or fresh—are a great addition to baked goods as these fruits are high in sugars but not as high as what you would use in the recipe. Play around to get a nice balance between fruit and sugar in your baked goods.

Just because you need to use honey a little less doesn't mean you have to give up flavoring your Greek yogurt. Apricots are high in fiber, vitamin C, and iron, and when you blend the fruit into a puree it can be added to your Greek yogurt—or even cream—to give that sweet tang you desire.

You can even create your own glazes using apple cider vinegar or balsamic vinegar. Balsamic vinegar isn't just made with the juice of grapes but rather the whole grape which includes the seeds, skin, and stem. The vinegar can be cooked down (reduced) until it becomes a sweet syrup that you can use to glaze whatever you wish.

Play around with all the tastes available to you. Sweet isn't the only flavor. Look to expand your palate with sour and bitter flavors so that you can remind your brain other tastes are just as great.

USING SWEETENERS IN BAKING

Not all sweeteners are equal in how they can be used. Some are better suited to cooking and baking while others are not. You will need to consider each carefully before sticking to a single choice or having several on hand for what you want to use them for.

Sugar replacement	Sweetener measurement	Sugar measurement	Recipe adaptations	Used for
Stevia	1 teaspoon	1 cup	The bulk of the recipe needs to be made up of extra butter, yogurt, or applesauce.	Baking and cooking.
Monk fruit	½ a cup	1 cup	None	Baking
Xylitol	1 cup of powder or ½ a cup of granulated xylitol.	1 cup	None	Good for cooking, baking, and browning.
Stevia in The Raw (stevia and erythritol)	½ a packet	1 teaspoon	Can't be used for caramelizing or browning. Not good for meringues. The temperature of the oven may need to be dropped by up to 25% for some recipes.	Baking
Sweet 'N Low (saccharin)	½ teaspoon or ½ a packet.	1 teaspoon	May create a lumpy texture.	Baking
Equal (aspartame)	½ a packet	1 teaspoon	Heat destroys sweetness so only use it for custards and cool puddings.	Use for cold puddings only.
Splenda (sucralose)	½ a packet or ½ a teaspoon.	1 teaspoon	Use Splenda baking formulation when baking.	Baking
Nectresse (erythritol)	½ a packet or ¼ teaspoon.	1 teaspoon	None	Baking
Coconut sugar	1 cup	1 cup	None	All
Honey	¾ cup	1 cup	None	All
Fruit concentrate (fruit juice with liquid removed)	¾ cup	1 cup	Reduce the liquid in the recipe by three tablespoons.	All
Maple syrup	¾ cup	1 cup	Reduce the liquid in the recipe by three tablespoons.	All

REPLACING SODAS

One of the largest contributing factors to ingesting high volumes of sugar is sodas. The reason people tend to choose sodas over other forms of drinks is that they are not only sweet but they tend to not be as boring. Luckily, there are many different ways to spice up your liquids so that you can enjoy them without any added sugar.

Water

Water may seem a little boring to have to drink but it should be your go-to drink when you are thirsty. Any additions to the water should make it more fun to drink for other occasions. You can add fruity flavors to water by creating infusions with your favorite fruits and spices. Next time you are craving some sugar, cut a few finger-length sticks of cucumber, get a few fresh mint leaves and a couple of blueberries, and leave them in a pitcher of water and ice for a few minutes before serving yourself a tall glass full. Fruit infusions are only limited by your imagination so play around with a wide variety of fruits to get the taste you want.

Soda Water

Some people struggle with giving up the feel of soda as well as the taste. Soda water should have no added sugars. Soda water can be made from home using products like Sodastream without adding the flavored syrups unless they are sugar-free. There are many things you can do with soda water. Add a touch of fruit concentrate—with no added sugar—to get the flavor of fruit you desire, or add slices of your favorite fruits to create a soda infusion. If you are missing lemonade then slice up a lemon or lime to add to your soda water with a sprinkle of your preferred sweetener to give you the sweet taste you desire.

Hot Drinks

Never discredit a cup of good green tea. It is jam-packed with antioxidants and can be enjoyed either hot or cold. It is virtually calorie-free unless you enjoy it with milk. Some of the benefits you will get when you drink green tea include lowering your risk of certain cancers, type 2 diabetes, obesity, and liver disease.

You can continue to drink coffee or regular tea with milk or whatever milk alternatives you prefer—ensuring that they are sugar-free—as long as you are monitoring your sweetener levels. The last thing you want to do is use the incorrect sweetener that results in problems for you.

Many herbal teas contain zero sugar but burst with all kinds of flavors. Combining hibiscus flowers with some cinnamon can result in a sour tea with a hint of sweetness you may enjoy. Play around with herbal tea combinations to find the one that best suits you.

Others

Pure fruit smoothies need to be switched for mostly vegetable smoothies as fruit tends to be far higher in fructose than vegetables. You can create your own antioxidant, mineral, and vitamin bursting concoction by playing around with various vegetable and fruit combinations.

If you are looking for something to hydrate you and replace electrolytes after a heavy training session look at using coconut water. This unique drink contains magnesium, sodium, potassium, and is very low in sugar. It is sure to help you with your recovery of sore muscles. Don't confuse it with coconut milk.

Kombucha is a fermented tea that is great for providing probiotics to your gut. This drink is an acquired taste. This product does contain a small dose of alcohol so, if you are sensitive to it or pregnant, then it is a better idea to give it a skip. This tea can be made from home or bought from a store. However, if you are buying from a store, ensure that you check the nutritional label to see if sugar has been added to it or not.

If you are someone who likes to add spirits to a preferred soda that is something that you will need to put a stop to. However, if you cannot give up alcohol try some red wine or other alcoholic drinks that contain no sugar. Remember to keep this in moderation and enjoy it occasionally.

SUGAR-FREE RECIPES

The following recipes are just to prove that you do not need added sugar to enjoy a dessert. These are by no means the only desserts available. Try these five recipes before you start collecting your own or experimenting by switching out the sugar of recipes you know for any alternative you feel comfortable using.

▷ *Apple Pie*

This recipe by Barbara is not keto-friendly—as apples are high in natural sugars—but there isn't any added sugar in this classic apple pie. Serve it with some cream or sugar-free ice cream as soon as it is out of the oven, or enjoy it cold.

Recipe Serving Size: 1 pie

Prep Time: 10 minutes

Cook Time: 45 minutes

Individual Serving Size: 1 slice, ⅛ of pie

Carbohydrates: 41.4 g

Sugar: 9.8 g

Protein: 3.1 g

Fat: 15.1 g

Calories: 308.6 kcal

Ingredients:

- Pastry for a 9-inch double-crust pie, sugar-free
- 12 oz apple juice concentrate, unsweetened
- 1 tbsp ground cinnamon
- 6 cups apples, thinly sliced
- 3 tbsp cornstarch

Directions:

- Preheat the oven to 350° F.
- In a small bowl mix the cinnamon, cornstarch, and ¼ of the apple juice.
- Then over medium heat, add the apple slices and the leftover apple juice to a saucepan then cook until the fruit is tender.
- Pour the cornstarch mixture into the saucepan and cook until the mixture starts to thicken.
- Pour the saucepan contents into the bottom of the pie crust then add the top. Decorate as you wish.
- Bake for 45 minutes.
- Remove from the oven and then serve.

▷ *Fluffy Chocolate Mousse*

This classic dessert is known to have a high sugar content which forces most dieters away. However, you do not need to desert this dessert thanks to Kim Lange. Enjoy this chocolaty treat with some fresh fruit feeling mostly guilt-free because it is so easy to make.

Recipe Serving Size: 4 servings

Prep Time: 5 minutes

Cook Time: 0 minutes

Individual Serving Size: ¼ of recipe

Carbohydrates: 7 g

Sugar: 1 g

Protein: 3 g

Fat: 21 g

Calories: 324 kcal

Ingredients:

- ⅓ cup cocoa powder, unsweetened
- 1 ½ cups heavy whipping cream
- ⅓ cup low-carb sweetener of choice, sugar-free

Directions:

- Add the heavy cream and sweetener to a bowl then use a hand mixer to thicken the mixture at a medium-low speed.
- Once the cream starts to thicken, add the cocoa powder and continue to beat until stiff peaks start to form.
- Divide among four serving bowls and serve immediately with your choice of berries.

▷ *Chocolate Chip Cookies*

Almost nothing is better than a chocolate chip cookie with some milk and, thanks to Christel Oerum, you can enjoy some sugar-free cookies whenever the need takes you. Remember to practice self-control as you don't want to use this recipe every other day.

Recipe Serving Size: 8 cookies

Prep Time: 5 minutes

Cook Time: 15 minutes

Individual Serving Size: 1 cookie

Carbohydrates: 9.4 g

Sugar: 0.4 g

Protein: 3.3 g

Fat: 14.3 g

Calories: 165 kcal

Ingredients:

- 3 tbsp ground flax meal
- 1 ½ cup almond flour
- 4 tbsp butter, softened
- 1 tsp baking soda
- ½ cup sweetener of choice, sugar-free
- 3 tbsp water
- ½ cup sugar-free chocolate chips
- Pinch of salt

Directions:

- Preheat the oven to 325° F.
- Line a baking tray with parchment paper.
- If using a granulated sweetener, blend it in a food processor until it is powdered. This should take about 10 seconds. Skip this step if you are already using a powdered sweetener.
- In a bowl add the softened butter and sweetener then mix until the sweetener is completely absorbed by the butter.

- Now add in the water, almond flour, ground flax meal, and baking soda then stir until all ingredients are well combined.
- Add the chocolate chips to the mixture and fold in until they are equally distributed.
- To make a single cookie you will need about one tablespoon of the dough. Scoop out the dough and arrange it on the lined baking tray.
- If you prefer a chewier cookie, cook for 16 minutes but if you prefer a cookie with more of a cake texture then cook for 19 minutes. They should be golden brown when they are ready.
- Remove from the oven and allow the cookies to cool for 10 minutes.
- Remove from the tray and add to a wire rack then let the cookies cool for another 10 minutes.
- The cooling step is important for if you don't do it the cookies will crumble apart.
- These cookies can last about a week in a sealed container.

▷ *Fudgy Brownies*

If you are a fan of brownies, then you simply cannot turn your nose up at Katrin Nürnberger's keto-friendly, low-sugar brownies. These delectable treats are so tasty you may need to give them away to prevent yourself from eating them all or freezing them.

Recipe Serving Size: 16 servings

Prep Time: 10 minutes

Cook Time: 25 minutes

Individual Serving Size: 1 square

Carbohydrates: 4.1 g

Sugar: 1 g

Protein: 2.9 g

Fat: 18.8 g

Calories: 192 kcal

Ingredients:

- 3 large eggs
- ¾ cup almond flour
- 6 oz butter unsalted, softened
- 6 oz dark chocolate, at least 85% (or sugar-free) and melted
- ⅓ cup cocoa powder, unsweetened
- ⅔ cup powdered sweetener, sugar-free

Directions:

- Preheat the oven to 355° F.
- Line a 5 x 9-inch baking tin with parchment paper so that the bottom and sides are covered.
- Using a heat-proof bowl add the blocks of chocolate then place the bowl into a pot that has boiling water to create a double boiler.
- You can melt the chocolate in the microwave but it needs to be at a low intensity and checked frequently to prevent the chocolate from burning. Melt in increments of 30 seconds or less until completely melted.
- Using a food processor blend together the softened butter, cocoa, powdered sweetener of choice, and eggs until fully combined.
- Then add the almond flour and melted chocolate then mix again until a thick yet smooth batter is made.
- Pour the batter into the lined dish and make sure the top is completely smooth.
- Bake for 25 minutes or until the top is starting to look solid.
- Allow the brownies to cool completely before cutting and removing them from the baking tray.

- Hot brownies are very soft and they need to cool down to allow them to firm up.

▷ *Vanilla Ice Cream*

Ice cream can be sugar-free and you do not need an ice cream maker to make your own delicious ice cream from The Sugar Free Diva.

Recipe Serving Size: 6 servings

Prep Time: 20 minutes

Freezing Time: 2.5–8 hours

Individual Serving Size: ⅙ of recipe

Carbohydrates: 6 g

Sugar: 4 g

Protein: 4 g

Fat: 29 g

Calories: 306 kcal

Ingredients:

- 2 tsp vanilla extract
- 2 cups heavy whipping cream
- ¾ cup powdered sweetener of choice, sugar-free

- 2 cups milk

Directions:

- If you do not have an ice cream maker then place the container you will be using in the freezer for at least an hour before you use it. Be sure to use a bowl that can be frozen safely. This step is not necessary if you are using an ice cream maker.
- Add all the ingredients to a blender and blend until well incorporated.
- If you are using an ice cream maker, add the ingredients to it and follow the instructions of the brand you are using.
- Otherwise, add the mixture to the frozen bowl and freeze it. Every 30 minutes, for the next two to two and half hours, you need to remove the bowl and beat the contents for a few minutes before placing it back into the freezer. Continue until the ice cream reaches the consistency that you prefer.
- Alternatively, you can get two Ziplock bags, one larger than the other. In the larger bag add ice and some salt. In the smaller one add some mixture from the blender. Add the sealed smaller bag to the larger bag before sealing the

larger bag and shake for about 10 minutes or until an ice cream consistency is reached. This could be a great activity for little kids as they can make their own dessert.

- You can add whatever flavors you want as long as they are sugar-free or you can simply add some of your preferred fruit.

Whether you are trying a keto diet or a sugar-free diet there are many different kinds of recipes you can try or adapt to your needs. There is no need to use added sugar in any recipe. The switch is possible, but you have to be willing to make it or it will never happen. Sugar-free foods may not have the necessary taste that you have gotten used to, but that just allows you to experiment with other flavors. Sweet isn't the only flavor available to you.

5

STOP BEING INFLUENCED FROM OTHERS

E ven once you decide to make a dietary change, you will find that many influences seem to get in the way of you achieving this. Some you will be in control of while others not so much. There are biological influences, such as your appetite and personal preference, that have an impact on what you eat or if you are hungry. Physical influences can include the time required to cook a good meal, your understanding of which foods are good for you or not, and the skills that you have to cook the meals that are good for you. You are constantly being influenced by the beliefs and knowledge you have about certain foods and the attitude you form to those foods. There is even a social influence where culture, meal patterns, and family can affect what and when you eat. These influences are those that you can do something about with some time, practice, and education about what you put on your plate. However, there are influences that you will struggle with trying to break away from, but you will need to do that to get away from the cycle of poor eating.

The first influence that can be a real challenge to break from is the economic influence. The cost of food, especially healthy food, isn't always as affordable as it should be when compared to less healthy foods. If your salary doesn't allow for you to eat more fresh fruits and vegetables weekly, it makes it more difficult to stick to a healthier diet than what one may assume. Generally the so-called "junk food" is sold at cheaper prices than healthier food. No wonder people are turning to those options instead of healthier foods. Lastly, there is the psychological influence of food. Eating certain types of food has a heavy influence on our moods and can trigger anything from pleasure to guilt, which can lead to stress.

HOW PSYCHOLOGY INFLUENCES YOU

When you are at home, you are in an environment that you can control. You decide what you bring into your home. However, the moment you step foot outside of your home, you are immediately bombarded with branding and advertising. Some people have an impact on your consumption of food and drink. Yet you cannot remain locked up in your home forever. You need to go out into the world and be with other people. You will need to learn to deal with the influences that are around you.

Color Psychology

Your brain has been conditioned for years to believe that certain colors are better than others. Companies who want to sell their products want them to stand out from their competition, so they use color psychology on their clients. Because of this fact, color is vital to the branding of a product. If the color doesn't match the expectations of the client then likely they will not buy the product at all.

People have been influenced by colors for decades if not for centuries. One of the most well-known occurrences is gender colors. Today, pink is considered a feminine color while blue is considered more masculine. However, these colors actually meant the opposite in the 19th century, resulting in blue being a delicate color meant for girls and pink being the color associated with strength and meant for boys. Before that, children weren't even assigned a color to denote their gender.

It is easy to manipulate the feelings of people using colors. Go on. Think of any color and you will have a feeling associated with it. Companies use this connection to sell more of their product regardless of the damage that they may cause.

Truthiness

Sometimes direct manipulation isn't needed to influence your brain into wanting something. Your brain perceives things a certain way if you are unaware of known facts. There is a good chance that you have assumed something to do with food that you believe is a fact due to the usage of certain colors, imagery, or photos that accompany the information you have been exposed to. You have no knowledge about this information but something in your gut leads you to believe that this is a true fact. This is known as truthiness.

Truthiness is the belief that something is real, yet can be partially or entirely false. Your brain can be influenced by many external sources to make certain products seem better to you in comparison to others. Think of the color red. Normally when one sees the color red it is interpreted as danger or a command being given i.e. a stop sign. Yet you also associate it with Valentine's day (and the consumption of chocolate) and even Christmas which is associated with Santa's red suit and people overeating during the holidays. So, if a product is decorated with the color red you may find that you are immediately attracted to it despite health concerns associated with the product. You may find yourself tempted to add it to your shopping cart. This is when your brain needs to break away from the influence and you have to check the nutritional contents so that you can make a factual decision about the product.

This influence is hardly limited to color but also imagery that involves people that you look up to. When you see a famous model or sports star drinking or eating something loaded with added sugars you immediately feel that since they are doing it surely it can't be that bad for you. Sadly, this is only your brain being tricked into buying different kinds of products. People who are in the limelight are paid to use those products by sponsors who then use that imagery in their advertising to sell to the general public. These images last longer than just a special on the product. Those images are retained in our memory and they will be revisited by the brain, again and again, therefore cementing a truthiness that is based on little to no fact. You end up forcing yourself to believe in half-truths.

Sadly, it is very easy to make a statement and believe it because it has a nice picture to go with it. But you need to learn to question these feelings of truthiness and replace them with well-known, well-researched facts.

This can only be done when you take the time to research the food that you eat and therefore learn to separate the true facts from the perceived facts.

HOW PEOPLE INFLUENCE YOU

From a very young age, you are taught that if you do not fit in you are an outcast and that there is something wrong with you. This mentality is carried over into your adult life where you seek the approval of everyone in a group situation, sometimes to your own detriment. When you are around certain people, friends, or family, you tend to adopt a type of behavior that best suits the group. This sort of behavior is neither good nor healthy and if you are trying to give up a sugar addiction it can be very difficult to do. Yet, how is it that a group can influence your decisions?

Whenever you make a decision you assign a certain value to it. For example, giving up sugar is the most important decision in your diet and so you attach more value to following it strictly. If more people within a group situation agree with you then you will find it easier to remain with your decision. However, if more people in your group are against the decision then the value of your decision diminishes while you are with that particular group. This can cause you to eat some sugar or even completely give up on your diet as there is no support from the group.

If the group goes out to eat at a restaurant and everyone orders one healthy meal you will be more confident in ordering similarly. Yet if you are the only one doing this, you are immediately singled out and end up feeling like an outsider with your own friends. The fear of being shunned due to one decision causes people to generally do as the group does to save face.

You lose your individuality once you are in a group and the majority vote will always win. "If everyone is eating dessert then so should I," becomes the thought that is in your brain. This behavior is due to humans' tendency to follow a group mentality as a way to be guided to the correct behavior. It is important to remember that this is rarely intentional on the group's part—unless they are a bunch of bullies, in which case you need better friends—as each person within the group is being influenced by another. This is a subtle kind of influence that you are not always conscious of and may even try to justify to outside people who are not part of the group and are therefore not influenced in the same manner. Typical excuses can be something to the effect of, "It was his birthday. Everyone else was eating cake. I just had to have a slice." By that reasoning, you can say that it isn't just about what and when you eat but also about who you eat with.

Social Modeling

When in a group situation—either with friends or complete strangers—you will look to those around you to see what the current social norms are. You will seek to imitate the group you find yourself in as best as possible even if it goes against your normal behavior. It becomes a situation of monkey see, monkey do. This prevents you from listening to the subtle cues—such as you may be full or don't want dessert—your body is trying to send you. There are different kinds of social modeling. There is impression management when you decide to eat a certain way because you want to give a certain kind of impression to the person or people you are eating with. Then there is social facilitation when you are eating more food because everyone around you is continually eating. This is seen most often at family gatherings that have no structured times and anyone can eat when they get hungry. Seeing other people eat makes you want to eat even after you have already eaten. This can lead to second helpings or mindlessly grazing on snacks that are provided. This can also work in reverse. If no one is eating you tend to not want to eat as well.

Why are social cues so effective? Likely because most people simply don't know any better. If someone gets up to have a second helping of food you may feel that it is alright to have a second helping as well. The same can be applied to having dessert. It makes saying no much more difficult, especially if it is a cake made by your grandmother who wants you to have a piece.

Yet group behavior is not always negative. If you have a group of friends who support your choices, they will encourage and help you reach your goals. They can work together to create group situations where you do not need to feel left out about your choices or force you to conform to what they are doing.

Even you by yourself can influence a whole group with the decisions you make. The group wants to conform, but there will always be individuals who are looking to others in the group to make moves so that they can follow. Instead of getting that second helping of potato salad or slice of cake, decide to have an ice-cold glass of your favorite infusion. Offer to make it for people and share with those that want to follow your behavior. Pretty soon, it may become the new social norm at your gatherings.

You can apply this behavior at home with your family, especially if you have impressionable youths under your care. If you are not providing them with healthy alternatives to junk food the members of your family are just going to continue the cycle of eating poorly. But if you take the time to add an extra vegetable or fruit into the meal plan, soon you will have family members eating more healthily. Be the change necessary for others to model themselves after a healthier person.

HOW TO AVOID NEGATIVE INFLUENCES

Dealing with negative influences can be as difficult as dealing with an addiction. Some of these influences can be internal and others are external. Although it will not be easy to deal with these negative influences, you will need to take charge of your life if you want to be happier with who you are now and in the future. You should start by surrounding yourself with positive people. Sadly, many people have the bad habit of remembering bad events—or negative things people have said to them—over and over in their heads. They do this for so long that they start to believe that it is true. Although it is a difficult task to do, you will need to root out these negative thoughts as they are poisoning you from the inside. If you have someone in your life who is constantly and consistently putting you down while trying to reinforce that you will never reach your goals, then you may have a negative person in your life.

It may not always be easy to recognize these kinds of people at first, but if you sit down and think about the people in your life, you may find that some exhibit nasty traits. They may not take accountability for anything they do. They always have to be correct, and if they can't be correct, they tend to play the part of the victim, especially if you call them out on their toxic behavior. They are controlling and manipulative in ways that you may not notice until you really think about their behavior toward you. These people may always need your help and expect you to drop everything yet if you are in the same position, they are nowhere to be found until they need help again. Lastly, and the most damaging of all, they do not respect any boundaries you put in place no matter how hard you try.

There are only two possible ways of dealing with these kinds of people. The first is to try and find balance by making the interactions with this person more positive. However, for some reason, certain people in your life are just negative people and are unwilling to change or double the effort to break you down. Then you are only left with one recourse. You will need to cut them from your life. This is easier said than done. If they happen to be an acquaintance it can be fairly straight forward and you just have to make an effort to avoid them. It becomes a lot more difficult if the negative person is a close friend or even a family member.

Some negative people are just impossible to cut out of your life. This is when you need to manage your time with them as well as your feelings toward them. Negative people will always be negative, but it is how you receive those negative comments and actions that can mean the difference between being able to shrug off the negative comment or allowing it to find a voice at the back of your mind. Try to not concentrate on their negativity but rather surround yourself with more people who are a positive influence on you. A weed can be choked out of existence if it isn't fed.

You are taking these steps because you deserve better than what these people are doing to you. Identify them and manage them as best suits you. Enforce boundaries and insist on them being respected. If these boundaries aren't respected then it is time to cut people from your life—but be sure that this is an action that is completely necessary before taking this step as it is irreversible. Remember, you are doing this for not only your physical health but also your mental health; you have no reason to feel guilty about wanting to be better. Allow the positive to outweigh the negative by not thinking of it all the time.

Negative people are external, but you can also be a negative and toxic influence on yourself. And sometimes it is easier to deal with those around you rather than yourself. However, you can do this. By setting out measurable and obtainable goals—keeping a journal or visual goals—you can set your sights on a brighter future. And when you have a bad day—and there will be bad days— you can look back on what you have achieved with positivity and encouragement. Never focus on the negativity of a day. Find something positive that happened during your day—even if it was a stranger smiling and giving you a friendly nod—and focus on that until all the negative feelings fade away. This way, even the smallest victory can carry you through the worst of days.

A lifestyle change may also be necessary, especially if there are negative aspects to your current habits. Changing an ingrained habit can be difficult and it may require someone a little stronger than you to manage it. Have a support system that you can rely on. Whether it is someone who can hold you accountable for your actions or someone you can call and talk with through the worst of your cravings, a solid support system made up of positive people is what will see you through this. Look for people who have gone through this before and pull them into your circle of influence. This is called association on purpose. People who have already managed to give up addiction to sugar can be a wealth of knowledge and advice. However, be prepared to hear some truths about yourself that you may not want to hear—no one likes to be called an addict—but are necessary. Don't see this as an attack on you but rather a piece of advice that can assist you with your goals.

HOW TO BE THE CHANGE NEEDED

This may not be an easy journey—as many people don't like change—but if it is subtle enough then, over time, they will change for the better. You cannot expect people to change their bad habits if you are not prepared to change yours. Lead by example so that you can be the person that people come to with questions or for advice. Raise awareness of healthier options for different kinds of meals. Be kind with the words that you use when you are trying to do this. Telling people they have to change their diet, because they will die if they don't, helps no one. There is no point in scaring people who may already be feeling guilty about the situation they find themselves in. Show people that the healthier options have been working for you in terms of health or even weight loss. People react better to kind words than threats.

If that doesn't seem to work then offer to cook for them. The quickest way to show people that there are foods that are better for them is to make quick, easy, nutritious meals that help with the diet they are following. But don't let them take advantage of you. Just when they start to get comfortable with your cooking, offer to teach them how to do it for themselves. Share tips and tricks that you have learned and part with some of your recipes so that others can also enjoy the meals that have been helping you with your healthier lifestyle. By encouraging this behavior many people in your life will start to cook better and healthier meals, which makes social gatherings so much easier to deal with.

If someone you know is going through the same thing as you, ask them if they would be willing to work together with you. This way, the two of you can be accountable to each other not only in what you eat but how you react in a group situation. This is a great way to prevent yourself, and someone else, from falling back on poor habits you are trying to give up. This help can extend beyond just the diet. Good behaviors can be made or broken by stress in a person's life. Help out when your accountability buddy wants to go to the gym or shopping without their children. Many sweet treats are marketed to children, so shopping with them can be a nightmare.

By helping others, you get people to understand that you are genuinely serious about becoming healthier. You also help people realize that you are willing to help them with their diet—which helps them to not feel alone in this endeavor—if they need it.

6

BE CONFIDENT AND MORE HAPPY

You are allowed to be happy, and don't let anyone —especially yourself—tell you the opposite! Once you manage to break away from sugar, poor habits, and negative influences you will be amazed at how your life will change for the better. Many aspects of your life will improve if only you stick to giving up sugar.

SUGAR DETOX

Although there are many benefits to giving up sugar, it just wouldn't be right to not discuss the disadvantages that will come from it. Once you decide to give up sugar, you will find that within the first few hours of not eating your usual sugary treat you are feeling great.

The need to have another treat isn't there by the end of the day, and by day two you're feeling full of energy despite not having any sugar. Then the end of day two or the start of day three hits you like a ton of bricks. You are in full-blown sugar withdrawal now and your brain is screaming at you to give it something sugary—and anything will do.

The brain isn't getting its dopamine or serotonin shots, your mood fouls, and you are very irritated with everyone around you. This state of transition will be difficult for most and feel near impossible for those that have been a slave to sugar addiction for several years. You will feel exhausted, suffer headaches, and even feel as if you cannot think straight. It will feel as if the end will never come; then a week passes and it all stops. You are over the worst of the withdrawal. This process can take anywhere from one week to several depending on the level of addiction, but within a month you should be completely free of sugar's hold on you. Eventually, your body will get used to the lowered glucose, serotonin, and dopamine levels; then your energy levels will start to increase. Even after a month, you should continue to avoid consuming any sugar. It is suggested that you give up sugar for at least a year before slowly allowing small amounts back into your life, but only if you want to!

To help with the sugar detox, plan your meals around good sources of protein—both plant and animal-based —and healthy fats with plenty of fiber from vegetables, grains, and fruits that are low in sugar. Try to avoid refined starches, such as bread, where you can as they do contain hidden sugars. Lower your intake of grain in favor of fiber-rich vegetables. Keep your fruit portions low while increasing your vegetable portions. Alcohol may impact the way you eat. If this does so negatively then it is a good idea not to drink alcohol while you are practicing mindful eating. It is best to give up alcohol— as it too will contain a lot of sugar—or drink it after the meal.

BENEFITS

Now that the negative part of breaking an addiction is out of the way, let's move on to the many benefits that you will be able to enjoy. Your energy levels will be more stable now as you will not get spikes in your blood sugar that disappear as quickly as they appear. With less blood sugar, your insulin is better managed, which causes a lowered risk of type 2 diabetes and lowers the amount of visceral fat that packs on around your middle. Less blood sugar also causes a drop in blood pressure which decreases the chance of heart conditions.

Inflammation can be triggered by sugar and when you are no longer consuming it your skin's condition starts to improve. This includes acne triggered by sugar as well as your complexion as the collagen and elastin start to strengthen once more. Once you are no longer suffering from chronic inflammation, your immune system gets a boost. With this boost, you will find that your health starts to improve because you are less likely to catch colds and flu.

Sugar also affects slow-wave sleep (SWS), which is required for you to sleep deeply and create memories. With less sugar in your life, the degree of SWS improves, which improves the consolidation of information learned during the day and creates a deeper sleep. This allows you to sleep through the night instead of waking up multiple times during your sleep cycle.

By not feeding sugar to the bacteria in your mouth, you will find your breath starts to improve and the occurrences of tooth decay diminish. Your brain will be more focused on tasks as it will no longer have that addiction that causes you to lose concentration in its need to get more sweet treats. Even your sex life will thank you for not consuming sweets. The sex hormones will return to the balance they are meant to be at, which will cause your libido to return to what it once was.

By cutting down the number of calories that you would be consuming with sugary goods you can start losing weight. However, to lose weight is more than just giving up sweets. Most people need only 2,000 calories to maintain their current weight, but if they want to lose weight they need to be in a deficit. This means that you need to be eating fewer calories than what your body needs in order to lose weight. A healthy way to do this is to reduce the number of calories you consume by 500. This will allow you to safely lose between one and two pounds a week. This is because one pound of body fat is 3,500 calories. By reducing your diet by 500 calories a day by the end of the week you will be in a deficit of 3,500 calories. By eating sugary and processed foods the calories you were consuming are often termed as "empty calories" which have little to no nutritional value but are high in calories. It becomes very easy to rack up calories while eating these types of foods. By replacing these foods with those that are nutrient-dense, high in protein, healthy fats, and fiber, dropping 500 calories a day is a lot easier.

Because of this, just giving up sugar isn't good enough to lose weight. You need a well-balanced diet that allows for a deficit of 500 calories a day or you will need to incorporate more exercise.

BUILDING CONFIDENCE

After years of addiction and suffering from negative comments—yours and from other people—your confidence is going to be nonexistent or very low. That doesn't mean that you can't build it up again. You need to just take one day at a time and work on yourself. To help keep building your confidence, you will need to learn to manage your stress before you can accomplish anything.

Stress

Stress causes people to run back to sugar time and time again. If you can manage your stress levels, especially when you are going through a sugar detox, you will be successful in giving up this vice. Stress is a natural occurrence and everyone suffers through it, though some handle it better than others. Stress is just your body's way of functioning in a fight-or-flight situation. What makes it so bad is that sometimes you cannot turn off your response to these stressful situations and you constantly feel the pressure with no relief. This chronic level of stress can cause several health issues that range from an elevated heart rate, increased blood pressure, to even stomach ulcers. Stress can be managed in a variety of ways and as long as you do not cope with your stress through emotional eating then this is already a step in the right direction.

If you only have a few minutes to yourself you can try either mantra meditation, mindfulness, or breathing exercises. When trying the mantra meditation you concentrate on a single thought, saying, or image and you focus all your attention on that until you feel calmer with the situation you are in. Sometimes your mind will want to wander to the stressful situation, but you should draw it back to what you have decided to focus on. Being mindful allows you to be aware of yourself, where you are, what you are doing, and what is going on with you. The focus should solely be on you and how you can break away from a stressful situation. Lastly, you can try breathing exercises to help you calm down or remain calm when under pressure. This practice only takes a few minutes and you can do it in your chair or you can find a place of solitude to try it. Take a four-second deep breath in through your nose and hold it for seven seconds before slowly letting it out over eight seconds. Repeat as many times as necessary to bring yourself the calm that you desire.

The next three options may take a little more time and you will likely feel more comfortable doing them in a place where you can fully relax and let go. The first of these techniques is autogenic training. This activity allows you to focus on the different parts of your body. Each time you think of a particular part of your body, say something nice about it. Say this aloud if you are comfortable doing so. Never say anything negative about yourself as it will only reinforce negative thoughts and will make it more difficult for you.

Then there is the progressive muscle relaxation technique. Take your time getting comfortable and take deep breaths where you fully extend and contract your stomach. Choose the muscles you want to start working with and contract them for five seconds before relaxing them for 30 seconds. You can start with whichever muscle group you want to first, but do try to go through all of them from the top of your head to your smallest toe. You can combine this technique with your breathing exercise to help you become more relaxed.

If you cannot go to a place that brings you the peace you need you will simply have to conjure the image yourself. With the use of guided imagery, you can picture yourself in a place that brings you the most inner peace. It isn't good enough to see this place in your mind's eye; you also need to envision the sounds you will hear and what you can smell. If you like, picture a scene from your life that has always brought you peace and stay with that image until you feel ready to return to reality.

There are several stress-busting activities that you can also do if you want to include such activity in a sedentary lifestyle. The first of these could be none other than yoga. This activity is great for strengthening muscles and helping with balance. The focus of this activity is posture and breathing. If you have never tried yoga before it is a good idea to go to a few classes to allow a professional to help you with the various poses. Start with the easier poses before trying some of the more complex and always remember to do a decent warm-up before starting.

Alternatively, you can try tai chi. Although this activity looks like it requires a lot of movement, you can just as easily do the movements sitting down as standing. This is the perfect activity for those that cannot stand long or are elderly. When practicing tai chi, you are fluidly moving from one pose to the next with graceful, dance-like movements. While you are doing this remember to concentrate on your breathing and enjoy.

Ultimately, you can do any form of exercise. Any exercise causes your brain to release endorphins and they make you feel great after a workout. This can be a good replacement for the dopamine-starved brain. Getting a buddy to go with you when you exercise for a good chat is an excellent way to deal with stress. The two of you can even brainstorm alternatives to helping with the stress you are feeling.

If you are looking for something a little less active then book yourself in for a massage. The combination of essential oils and massage is sure to calm you down and allow you to focus on the task at hand instead of the stresses involved. Perhaps you don't like people to touch you and that's okay. There are other ways to relax. Fill a bath with hot water and add a few drops of essential oil to give yourself an aromatherapy session. If you prefer to shower, get some fresh herbs to hang in the shower to enjoy the same effect. You can also apply aromatherapy to your bedtime routine. You do this by adding a few drops to a diffuser or a few drops to your pillow so that you can breathe it in as you read a book or fall asleep. When choosing a scent, pick one associated with relaxation—something like lavender—or at the very least a scent that makes you feel relaxed.

You can even use music or art to help you express your feelings of stress and work through them. Not all the methods are foolproof and it is up to you to decide which best suits you. Just remember to choose an activity that doesn't cause more stress than it relieves.

Exercise

When you think of exercise, you may think of someone who is running for miles at a stretch without breaking a sweat. This is but one form of exercise, one which has taken years, if not decades, to achieve. There are different kinds of exercise that you can try to help with managing your stress or accompanying your weight loss journey. If you are not sure where to start, then it is best to try a little of everything to see which type of exercise suits you. Exercise can be broken down into three categories: strength, flexibility and balance, and cardio (aerobic and anaerobic) exercise.

For strength training, you can use free weights—like those you see in the gym—or you can use your own body weight. Exercises that revolve around this kind of training include push-ups, sit-ups, and squats. Or you can use weights to train individual muscles.

Exercises like tai chi and yoga are for people who want to concentrate on their flexibility and balance. These exercises are crucial to building a stronger body. If you are not flexible enough then there is a chance you will injure yourself while trying any form of exercise. This is why a warm-up session is required before training to allow the muscles to stretch and become supple before they are worked hard. The balance aspect of exercise is important to individuals who are likely to fall and injure themselves seriously. By improving your balance, you not only manage to keep on your feet when you stumble but the smaller muscles in your body get trained more regularly.

Although strength, flexibility, and balance exercises are very important to the body, the most important is likely the aerobic exercises. Although many people refer to this as cardio training this is actually inaccurate. Cardio training involves the heart pumping harder to circulate more oxygen to the rest of the body but it takes on two forms. When you are training and you are breathing so hard that it requires you to take a break to catch your breath then you are doing anaerobic exercise. Not many people can achieve this and keep going at it for an extended period as it requires a certain amount of fitness to achieve. It should also be done for short periods.

If you are the kind of person to start exercising for the first time, you should concentrate on aerobic forms of exercise first. This will help you build up the stamina and fitness to reach those higher goals. Aerobic exercise gets the heart pumping—similar to that of anaerobic exercise—but it doesn't hit a peak where you are gasping for breath. You should have elevated breathing and heart rate but should never have to stop what you are doing because you are gasping for breath. Aerobic exercise is great for you as it helps to improve fitness as well as benefits you mentally and physically. Although there are several types of equipment you can buy to do aerobic exercise with, there is no need for that; you do not even need a gym membership. Walking, cycling, swimming, and even hiking count as aerobic exercise.

You can start out small—as you will need to train your body to take on later challenges—something as simple as walking for five minutes before turning around and returning is 10 minutes worth of exercise. This time and the speed at which you do it at (intensity) can be increased every time you feel it is getting too easy. Over several weeks you will find that your fitness improves and you can walk or even run farther distances.

The important thing to remember is that you need to choose an exercise that you enjoy doing. If you hate doing a certain exercise, you will have no reason to keep doing it. If you find that exercising is difficult to get into or simply boring, find a way to distract yourself while you are doing it. Listening to your favorite album while you walk, or cycling through your favorite binging series—on a stationary bike—gives you between 30 and 60 minutes worth of exercise and helps you to pass the time. Many places—not necessarily a gym—offer classes in certain types of exercise. Go to these classes and ask for advice while a professional determines what level of difficulty you can comfortably do. This way, you can discover if you like a particular type of exercise as well as ensure you do not pick up an injury.

How often you exercise is up to you, though it is encouraged to do at least 30 minutes of exercise most days of the week, if not every single day. Before you say that you do not have 30 minutes to spare, you do not have to do 30 minutes concurrently. Break it into three sections of ten minutes each and divide it across your whole day. By doing this you not only get your 30 minutes a day but it prevents you from sitting too long in one place. Alternatively, you can try a continuous exercise that lasts for 20 to 60 minutes for at least three days a week. Take an hour-long walk, at a moderate pace, to explore new places and meet up with a friend for a chat.

By doing aerobic exercise often, you train your heart to pump more blood per beat. This will allow for a great volume of blood carrying oxygen to get to the muscles that need it to work properly. The more effort you put into your training the less often your heart will need to pump; your heart is, after all, a muscle that also needs training. As the blood will be carrying more oxygen to the muscles, they are less likely to become starved of oxygen, making it easier to train for longer periods.

With more oxygen, your body can also burn more calories and more calories burned means a higher deficit which allows you to lose extra weight.

Exercise, in general, has been proven to help with the risk of type 2 diabetes, lowers the risk of cardiovascular diseases, lowers high blood pressure, and aids in weight control and obesity management. You can even lower the risk of certain cancers such as those that develop in the colon and breast tissues. Bone density is better in those who exercise than those who don't. All it takes is 30 minutes a day—10 minutes in the morning, 10 minutes at lunchtime, and 10 minutes before dinner. It is that simple.

SELF-CONFIDENCE AND ITS IMPORTANCE

You aren't born with self-confidence. Your confidence is shaped by those around you. If you have people in your life that are supportive and give guidance, you are likely to develop a healthy level of self-confidence. However, if you are surrounded by people who are negative or overbearing, you will tend to develop lower self-confidence. This results in you being unable to make a decision or always second-guessing yourself.

Self-confidence is the feeling you get when you absolutely trust in yourself in every way possible. When you have self-confidence you believe that you can do anything. Sadly, many people tend to have very low self-confidence due to many different reasons. This doesn't mean that it has to stay low. Self-confidence ebbs and flows depending on what is influencing you. If you are surrounded by negative thoughts and actions you will lose self-confidence, whereas if you are surrounded by positive influences, you will grow your self-confidence.

It isn't only external factors that play a role in your self-confidence. You play a role too. If you are continually putting yourself down, your self-confidence will suffer. It becomes a vicious cycle that can be difficult to break away from. If you believe in your ability to do something then you are likely to try your best to achieve it. But if you talk yourself down, insisting that you can't do it, you won't even try to do it in the first place. You can't fail if you don't try, right? Wrong. It is the worst kind of failure because you convinced yourself of your inability to do it without even trying.

Thoughts have a powerful impact on what we can and can't do—but they are not alone. Convincing yourself to do something is but a small part of a whole. Once you have convinced yourself of wanting something you need to put a plan into action and then put a lot of effort into the plan. Sometimes a little talent can help this along. These various aspects are what need to come together for you to be able to build up your self-confidence to do something successfully. However, it all starts with you believing in yourself.

So you want to give up sugar. You have thought of it countless times but now you have a plan. Put that plan into action and really apply yourself to creating healthy meals while ignoring sugar. You may even find that you have some talent for cooking and creating many different kinds of sugar-free dishes, or perhaps you get really good at ignoring the negative people in your life who are trying to break down your self-confidence. Breaking an addiction is difficult but it is not impossible when your self-confidence is high. It actually becomes quite manageable the more effort and consistency you put into it.

However, all of this seems impossible when your self-confidence has been trampled again and again. Fear not, for you can do something to help boost your self-confidence and take back the power in your life. It will take some time, and you will need to put some effort in, but it is completely possible. The first thing that you need to work on is improving your self-efficacy. You need to truly believe in yourself. This journey you are setting out on is possible and you can do it. You have all the information at your fingertips to achieve your goals. Keep these positive thoughts with you as they are there to help you persist in your task despite facing possible setbacks.

Next, you need to work on increasing your self-esteem. You need to believe that you are important enough to yourself and others. You have as much right as everyone else to exist and be happy. This can be boosted by those around us as well as through achievements we accomplish, even if they are small.

The last is probably the hardest one to work on as it is trying to have a positive self-image. The reality is that we are being bombarded with a perceived standard of beauty and fitness that almost no one can achieve. Because of this, you may not be happy with the way you look now, but this will all change when you drop sugar from your life. You will start to feel better and in time your body will follow suit. By perceiving yourself in a better light, you will find that your self-confidence and self-esteem will improve. Just remember to avoid negative people who try to drag you down. What matters is you and how you feel about yourself. Don't let other people's venom infect you.

Write down messages to yourself to help with these three points or even create mantras that help you get through the day. Some days will be easier than others, so be sure to change any negative things you want to say to yourself to something more positive. This way you grow your self-confidence despite what other people do to you. When you are exuding self-confidence you can infect those around you! If you are in a leadership position this is a sure way to help lead those that work with you. Perhaps you can even encourage the replacement of the poor snacks in your cafeteria with healthier choices.

7

CONSISTENCY IS THE KEY

Giving up sugar for 24 hours is great for you, giving it up for life can be a daunting task. You will need to form some new habits around the types of food you eat. Forming a new habit can take between 18 and 254 days (Frothingham, 2019). For this habit to become something that you do automatically you need on average 66 days. Assuming you eat five small meals a day, you will need to make 330 meal choices that exclude sugar and other processed meals. This consistent behavior is what is going to help you end your addiction. You will not be able to succeed in your health and diet if you do not show consistency.

Consistency is the ability to do or believe in something for an extended period that will in the end be of some benefit to you. However, as seen, consistency is something that takes time and requires great patience. When you start this journey, you will not be able to see how your life will benefit in the end. But once you have completed those 330 meal choices, you will be able to look back and realize that it was worth it. It also requires great dedication and commitment as it is simply a repetition of a good eating habit until you achieve what you set out to achieve.

WHY CONSISTENCY IS NEEDED

By being consistent in your desire to not consume sugar, you cause people to react to your choices in a hopefully positive manner. They know that you don't eat sugar so they stop offering it to you and become part of your support system. By remaining consistent you can not only reach your health goals, but you can break away from the destructive addiction to sugar. By being healthier you are not only adding years to your life, but you are also building up your self-confidence which leads to a more successful life.

By being more consistent in your actions you will see problems that may stand in your way and deal with them before they become something you can't handle alone. You will develop trust in yourself to be able to handle these problems successfully. This will cause your goals to become more achievable and your progress toward your final goal becomes easier to handle. By remaining consistent in your actions, you become accountable for everything you do, the good and the bad included.

Because of this, you develop and improve your self-control by making disciplined decisions. You know that there is a goal that needs to be achieved and what you need to do to achieve it. By being consistent in one part of your life you can learn to be consistent in other parts of it, not just health but also with your finances or relationships.

WHY CONSISTENCY FAILS

There are several reasons that consistency could fail. The first is that humans have long been trained to want instant gratification and when they cannot have it they give up on trying to achieve something. As there is no patience to wait for the good to happen, people often give up before the benefits of their actions are seen. At other times the focus on the task at hand isn't there and so it becomes too difficult to maintain. Then, many people believe that if they cannot have their goal it isn't worth even trying for. Lastly, if there is no support to help with the consistency of a task then the task will simply stop.

By taking the time to be consistent you are not only learning new habits (such as surviving without sugar) but also new skills (cooking or baking) and building yourself up for a long, successful, healthy life. Day one is but one step and, though it may be difficult, by the time you reach day 66 you will look back at the first day and realize how far you have come. Consistency allows you to grow and improve as a person.

HOW TO PRACTICE CONSISTENCY

The first step is to have a plan that you can put into action. This plan needs to be well documented and something you can refer back to for the goals you want to achieve. Avoid making your plan flashy and requiring instant results; remember that this will take time. Set many smaller goals that can be consistently achieved with some effort on your part. Don't be idle if you have any spare time. Keep growing your knowledge through research and discovering new recipes or start getting more active with many different kinds of exercise. And if a slip-up occurs, treat it as a learning opportunity and not a disaster. The quicker you can bounce back from a slip-up the quicker your consistency can restart.

Consistency and Diet

Being consistent will help you achieve what is needed in your new healthy lifestyle but it can be boring due to the constant repetition. When something is boring you may want to deviate from your set plan, and this can cause you to lose the consistency that is needed to break an addiction. To prevent this from happening, you may have to implement a few steps to help you get back on track with your plan.

The first is to ask yourself why you believe consistency will help you with your endeavors. Draw up a list of pros and cons with eating sugar in mind and then compare the results. Use the first chapter of this book if you have forgotten how detrimental sugar is to your health. Having this visual aid will help you when those cravings start to hit. Keep it with your journal or a place that you often look at, such as your fridge or pantry, so that you can be reminded from time to time why you are doing this in the first place.

Be ready to deviate from your plan if it becomes necessary. There is a likelihood that something may disrupt your plans—such as an invitation to dinner when you didn't have time to prepare something for yourself—which can cause a disruption to the consistency you have been working so hard on. By being prepared to change your plan a little, you can react positively and not punish yourself for what has happened. By having knowledge about certain foods, you can make a choice with what you should and shouldn't eat at a surprise dinner. You can turn down foods or simply eat them in moderation to help overcome this. As long as you return to the plan of action with the next meal, you have lost nothing and gained a better understanding of controlling your eating habits.

The last thing to help you with your consistency is to know when you have outgrown your original plan. A routine is only good if you are benefitting from it in some way. When you are no longer benefitting from the plan that you have set in motion, then it is time to change it so that it does benefit you. Or perhaps you have already reached your goal and would like to reintroduce your favorite treat back into your life. However, you are not prepared to have to deal with the addiction to sugar once more. Change your plan to help you with new goals you want to achieve. You have the power to tweak your plan as you see fit. As long as you are benefitting and still striving for a goal, that is all that matters.

How to Be Consistent On Your Plan

Once you have decided on your plan of action and determined your goals—this plan needs to be something that you can stick to for a long period—you will need to clear your home of all sugary treats and processed meals. Box these up and give them away or, alternatively, finish the treats over time and do not replenish them when you go shopping. However, it is better to draw the line and stop immediately than try to wean yourself off of sugar slowly.

Once these foods are out of your house, go through your cupboards and fridge while educating yourself about what is in the food in the boxes, cans, and bottles. If there is anything that contains high concentrations of sugar get rid of it as well. This is the perfect time to reorganize your storage areas. Wash the cupboards and fridge before returning the food that you want to keep. Think of this as a symbolic gesture of cleansing yourself of the poor diet of the past.

Put together a meal plan for a week that includes all main meals as well as several snack options per day. Aim for meals that use ingredients that are fresh and nutrient-dense while avoiding using too many processed goods. Know what you want to include and what you want to avoid in your new diet and lifestyle. Always keep this in the back of your mind as you are going through recipes and designing your meal plan. If you are not comfortable doing this by yourself go speak with a registered dietician or nutritionist.

Once that is completed, sit down and draw up a shopping list of different kinds of foods that will be needed for the meal plan you have looked at. This will not only be your guide, but you can set up the list in such a way that you can avoid areas in the store where your favorite treats lurk. Only go to the aisles that contain the foods that are on the list to avoid any temptation. Another useful tip is that you should never go shopping when you are hungry. Your brain is going to try and convince you to get some food that can provide it with quick energy. These are the foods that you want to avoid.

Know what you are putting into your body. Whenever you are looking at foods in the store be sure to check the nutritional information as well as the ingredient list to know exactly what is in them. Try to limit the number of processed foods that you are buying, but if it is unavoidable then choose the whole-grain varieties for your baked goods or pasta varieties.

When adding items to your cart, concentrate on not only the macronutrients—protein, fat, and carbohydrates—but also the micronutrients such as minerals and vitamins. A great way to get the micronutrients you need is by eating a wide variety of vegetables and fruit. Don't just limit yourself to a single color. The more colors you consume the better! Try up to five different colors a day, as this is a sure way to not only get the fiber and water you need but also different kinds of phytochemicals, antioxidants, vitamins, and minerals. When choosing your fruits and vegetables try to stick to those that are in season and have not been stored away in cold storage. By eating seasonal fruits and vegetables you are getting the best benefits for the season. Citrus fruits—such as grapefruit or lemons—are more readily available during winter than other fruits. They provide you with boosted vitamin C to help your immune system with those seasonal colds and cases of flu.

Don't eat what you don't like! There are always alternatives to different food types. If you don't like spinach then don't use it in your recipes. Look to other vegetables such as kale or arugula for the recipe, and if being used in a salad use either romaine or iceberg lettuce. The possibilities are endless if you take the time to do the research. Explore all possible alternatives to replace foods that you do not like to eat with those that you do.

Once you have the habit of shopping only for what you need for your diet, and you do not deviate from it for several weeks, then you are well on your way to beating your addiction. However, don't forget to listen to what your body is telling you every step of the way. When you are hit with a craving, think about why this craving is there, but don't allow yourself to crave anything. This may seem a little counterintuitive—considering how you would normally ride out a craving instead of giving into it—but there is a reason for this. A craving is still your body's way of telling you that it needs something. Is your craving for chocolate cake or is it the taste of chocolate that you miss? Find alternatives to what you are craving so that you can ease the transition away from sugar. Think your cravings through to discover what your body truly needs at that moment. There is always wiggle room when consistency is needed on a plan.

Eat your meals consistently. Unless you are practicing a fasting technique, there is no reason for you to ever skip a meal. Make sure that each meal that you do eat is made up of all the macronutrients that are needed. The more nutrient-dense a meal is, the less hunger and cravings you will feel. You do not have to have three massive meals a day. By breaking your main meals into smaller meals that you can eat throughout the day you stave off feelings of hunger that could trigger cravings. Never allow yourself to feel starved as this can cause you to overeat when you eventually do have a meal. Always eat in moderation. Never overdo one thing in your diet as it can cause a well-balanced diet to become skewed and lead to other problems that can have an impact on your health.

Don't forget to hydrate! This is the quickest way to help you determine if you are dehydrated, hungry, or have a perceived hunger driven by boredom. Water doesn't have to be boring so spice it up with fruit or get unflavored, unsweetened soda water to quench your thirst. Always carry water with you wherever you go so that you can quench your thirst and check if you are truly hungry or not.

If possible, avoid eating out as this will help lower the chance of encountering foods that you have decided to give up. Concentrate on making more home-cooked meals so that you know exactly what is in the food you are placing on your plate. To ensure that there are always healthy meals ready for you when you get home, practice the art of food prepping. Cooking several types of meals when you have the time to do so allows for you to have a meal ready for the days that you do not have time to prepare. Although most cooked food shouldn't be stored in the fridge for more than three to five days—depending on what kind of food it is—many recipes can be frozen for much longer before they are used. Bulk cooking meats and grains before portioning them is a great way to ensure you have a meal either in the fridge or ready to be defrosted at any minute.

Always have snacks ready to go. What you have is only limited by your dietary constraints and your imagination. Create snacks the same way you would prep your meals and store them away so that they are never far from your reach when you need them. You can even create your own condiments and dipping sauces that can go with your snacks if you so wish.

Now you have a solid base to help you with the consistency of eating the same types of meals throughout your plan. However, these are not the only things you will need to practice. You will also need to learn how to avoid things that can distract you. Don't get caught up in new fad diets and food plans that promise you results that are never guaranteed. Jumping around from diet to diet can cause you to lose focus on the plan you have in place, and can jeopardize what you have already achieved and what you could achieve in the future. If you find that you are losing focus, try some new recipes or talk to the people in your support group to help you return focus to your plan.

Be mindful of not only what you eat but also of your activities such as exercise or meditations. Do this at a moderate level as often as possible—before trying more intense levels—to get all the benefits associated with your chosen activities. Never overdo exercise, as that is the quickest way to quit before you can enjoy all the benefits. Design a regimen that works for you; not everyone is capable of getting a mile run in before 6 a.m., just as not everyone can spend 30 minutes during a lunch break doing some relaxing yoga or tai chi.

Don't obsess over your weight needing to go down immediately once you start a diet. It took a while to gain the weight and it may take a while for you to lose it. Don't rely on a single type of measurement to judge your progress and success. Weight can fluctuate, losing inches can stall, and biomarkers can remain unchanged. Sometimes nothing happens for several weeks and this is where your consistency may crumble because you are not getting any results. If you honestly believe your plan is no longer working then change it, but don't ever give up. You have supportive people you can rely on and you can always speak to your physician about what could be preventing you from gaining the health benefits of not eating sugar.

Have coping mechanisms in place for when days are really bad. Speak to those that support you, update your journal, do a lot of meal prep, but at all costs avoid binging on sugar. As long as you are distracted from the so-called "need" for sugar you will forget it in time. However, it is important not to replace one addiction with another, so be sure to have healthy coping mechanisms that pave the way to your final goal.

If all else fails in keeping you focused on your plan, then look back to the diseases that are caused by the excess use of sugar. You may be the kind of person that desperately needs to quit sugar, and though it is better to not feel pressured into doing something, sometimes it is necessary to keep you from making a bad choice. You are not just doing this for yourself but also for those around you. By setting a good example, you become the person that someone else may need in their life to decide to finally break away from an addiction. Not only that, but you may be the person that encourages your whole family to eat better and destroy the notion that some diseases run in the family rather than being caused by terrible eating habits.

No one but you is in charge of your health. No one can force you to go on a diet or to cut certain foods from what you eat. This choice starts and ends with you. When you make the conscious decision to change your life you are literally taking your life into your hands and changing it for the better. Set a good example and add years to your life instead of slowly wasting away from an illness that could be prevented. You owe it to yourself.

CONCLUSION

Sugar, in some form or another, has been around since before humans. And once humans got a taste for it, that was that. In the past, sugar made the world go round, but now all it does is make you round! Sugar can be found in many different kinds of foods and drinks. Sometimes the addition of sugar is obvious when you check the list of ingredients, yet other times it hides under different names. It can easily do this because sugar has over 50 different names for the same destructive compound. Sugar is used not only as a sweetener for a variety of goods but also provides structure to baked goods. It is in practically everything that is edible.

Because of the tendency for sugar to be in many kinds of foods, especially in heavily processed, ready-made meals and sauces, you have likely been consuming it both knowingly and unknowingly for years. If you are someone who has always managed to keep their sugar eating habits to a moderate level you likely have not noticed any detrimental effects on your body. However, if you are someone who has never bothered to control your sugar intake you may have noticed that you are suffering. This is because excessive eating of sugar leads to illnesses such as type 2 diabetes, weight gain, obesity, high blood pressure, and even several types of cardiovascular diseases. Even if the hidden diseases haven't progressed enough for you to see the results, there are many other symptoms that you should not ignore.

By eating too much refined sugar you are damaging your teeth, skin, and most of your internal organs. Even your brain isn't left unscathed. When you eat sugars your brain reacts by releasing dopamine which activates the pleasure center in your head. This makes you feel good about eating sugar and want more. When you stop eating sugar the brain becomes deprived of the dopamine and it starts demanding that you feed it more sugar. Sugar has been noted as being as addictive as heroin and almost as difficult to give it up. You may already be addicted to sugar and not even know it yet!

Fear not, though; you do not have to remain addicted to sugar. There is a way to break away from it, but it will require you to have the strength and willpower to do so. The first step to getting over an addiction is admitting that you have a problem. Once that is out of the way and you remain honest with yourself, you can start to think about how you will overcome this hurdle in your life. You will need to dedicate some time to thinking of a plan that allows for you to not only enjoy your life but to do so without sugar through the use of alternatives.

You do not need to eat sugar as it doesn't contribute to your survival. By replacing sugar with different alternatives you will find that you never needed sugar in your life to begin with. There are many kinds of alternatives that you can use and you need to go through each of them to see which best suits you. Giving up sugar doesn't mean that you cannot enjoy the taste of all your favorite desserts. Thanks to diets such as the Paleo, Atkins, and the keto diet, there are many recipes online that can help you overcome a sweet tooth that is addicted to sugar. Sugar has long been associated with sweetness, but as you play around with a variety of sweeteners you will find that you can make do without it.

However, even with diets and recipes dedicated to eating less sugar, you may find that you are still craving that sweetness. The brain loves sugar because of the dopamine response that it causes and this is one of the physical attachments to sugar that you will need to break before you can hope to get over your addiction. Dealing with a physical addiction can take some time to do, but it is possible. However, you will never be free of a physical addiction if you do not deal with any emotional attachments you may have to sugar. Sugar has long been used as comfort food and you have likely grown accustomed to using it to deal with feelings of loss, loneliness, and even trauma. Once the emotional attachment to sugar has been broken, you will find that it becomes easier to deal with the physical attachment. This will help you to get over the cravings and withdrawal symptoms that you will be suffering.

While battling against sugar addiction, you will find that people and places will influence your ability to do this successfully. Don't allow yourself to be surrounded by people who tell you that you are not strong enough to beat this addiction. This will only result in more emotional cravings for sugary treats. Work on getting more positive people in your life to help you form a strong, positive support group. These are going to be the people to whom you will need to turn to when you feel at your lowest. This journey is going to be tough, but by having a strong support group you will have people who you can rely on to help you.

The key to dumping sugar once and for all is your confidence and being consistent in what you do. Poor diets usually result in a poor self-image that directly affects your confidence. By giving up sugar, your body will change for the better which will lead to a better self-image and contribute to having more confidence. Don't allow stress to erode your newfound confidence. Stress can be dealt with in many ways from self-care to trying a new form of exercise. These distractions will not only help you by distracting you from the sugar cravings but also help you create a calorie deficit. This deficit is needed if you want to lose weight. By staying on your plan to give up sugar and repeating it for every meal you will find that in due time even the worst of the cravings start to diminish before they eventually fade away.

By reading this book from cover to cover you have gained the knowledge to make the change to get away from sugar. However, knowledge is not enough. You need to apply this knowledge to your own life to get the benefits from a diet with no sugar. No book in the world can force you to do this. You are the one with the power and this book only provides you with some advice. Take that advice and use it to create a better you. Be the person who can be looked up to as an example of someone that tore themselves away from addiction and not only survived but still thrives. All you have to do is make a choice. So go on, choose to give sugar up today for a better, healthier you. You have the strength to do this.

BIBLIOGRAPHY

Anthony, M.-C. (2018, August 27). *The power of being consistent.* MC's Perspective. https://www.mariechristinanthony.com/blog/the-power-of-being-consistent

Barbara. (n.d.). *No-Added-Sugar apple pie.* Allrecipes. https://www.allrecipes.com/recipe/13859/no-added-sugar-apple-pie/

Barnwell, A. (2018, December 3). *Secret sugars: The 56 different names for sugar.* Virta Health. https://www.virtahealth.com/blog/names-for-sugar

Beres, L. (2019, May 7). *A guide to baking & cooking with 10 healthy sweeteners.* Earth911. https://earth911.com/home-garden/cooking-baking-with-healthy-sweeteners/

Blain, J. (2016, June 1). *Self confidence – the key to happiness, fulfilment and success.* Www.linkedin.com. https://www.linkedin.com/pulse/self-confidence-key-happiness-fulfilment-success-blain-game-changer/

Boyers, L. (2019, May 20). *How many teaspoons of sugar are there in a can of coke?* Livestrong.com https://www.livestrong.com/article/283136-how-many-teaspoons-of-sugar-are-there-in-a-can-of-coke/

Braverman, J. (2019, May 3). *How much weight can I lose if I eliminate sugar?* LIVESTRONG.COM. https://www.livestrong.com/article/525151-how-much-weight-can-i-lose-if-i-eliminate-sugar/

CDC. (2021, April 5). *Childhood obesity facts.* Centers for Disease Control and Prevention. https://www.cdc.gov/obesity/data/childhood.html

Cooke, S. (2016, October 27). *9 ways to say no to sugar.* The Alternative Daily. https://www.thealternativedaily.com/how-to-cut-out-sugar/

DiGiulio, S. (2020, January 8). *6 really good things that happen to your body when you quit sugar.* Health.com. https://www.health.com/nutrition/health-benefits-quitting-sugar

Edermaniger, L. (2019, August 30). *Carbs vs sugar: What's the difference and why it matters.* Atlas Biomed Blog. https://atlasbiomed.com/blog/carbs-vs-sugar-what-is-the-difference/

Editor. (2017a, May 5). *High blood pressure: Why excess sugar in the diet may be the culprit.* Diabetes. https://www.diabetes.co.uk/in-depth/high-blood-pressure-excess-sugar-diet-may-culprit/

Editor. (2017a, May 5). *High blood pressure: Why excess sugar in the diet may be the culprit.* Diabetes. https://www.diabetes.co.uk/in-depth/high-blood-pressure-excess-sugar-diet-may-culprit/

Editor. (2017b, May 15). *The harm of sugar: Why health risks should be compared to alcohol.* Diabetes. https://www.diabetes.co.uk/in-depth/harm-sugar/

Eenfeldt, A. (2021, July 1). *Keto sweeteners - the visual guide to the best and worst.* Diet Doctor. https://www.dietdoctor.com/low-carb/keto/sweeteners

Erdman, S. (2021, April 9). *Relaxation techniques: Learn how to manage stress.* WebMD. https://www.webmd.com/balance/features/blissing-out-10-relaxation-techniques-reduce-stress-spot

Eske, J. (2019, May 31). *Does insulin make you gain weight? Causes and management.* Www.medicalnewstoday.com. https://www.medicalnewstoday.com/articles/325328

EUFIC. (2006, June 6). *The factors that influence our food choices.* Eufic.org. https://www.eufic.org/en/healthy-living/article/the-determinants-of-food-choice

Felman, A. (2019, November 6). *Health risks of coca-cola: What it does to the body.* Www.medicalnewstoday.com. https://www.medicalnewstoday.com/articles/297600

Frothingham, S. (2019, October 24). *How long does it take for a new behavior to become automatic?* Healthline. https://www.healthline.com/health/how-long-does-it-take-to-form-a-habit

Garvey, K. K. (2009, July 28). *First native american honey bee.* ANR Blogs. https://ucanr.edu/blogs/blogcore/postdetail.cfm?postnum=1544

Gowin, J. (2011, August 8). *7 reasons we can't turn down fast food.* Www.psychologytoday.com. https://www.psychologytoday.com/za/blog/you-illuminated/201108/7-reasons-we-cant-turn-down-fast-food

Grannan, C. (2019). *Has pink always been a "girly" color?* Encyclopædia Britannica. https://www.britannica.com/story/has-pink-always-been-a-girly-color

Guerra, J. (2019, February 15). *What happens to your body and brain when you stop eating sugar.* Insider. https://www.insider.com/what-happens-when-you-stop-eating-sugar-2019-2

Guo, K. L. (2008). DECIDE: A decision-making model for more effective decision making by health care managers. *The Health Care Manager,* 27(2), 118–127. https://doi.org/10.1097/01.hcm.0000285046.27290.90

Harvard Health Publishing. (2019, November 5). *The sweet danger of sugar.* Harvard Health. https://www.health.harvard.edu/heart-health/the-sweet-danger-of-sugar

Hersheyland. (2020, December 30). *6 sweet sugar substitutes for baking.* https://www.hersheyland.com/stories/6-sweet-sugar-substitutes-for-baking.html

Howard, J. (2017, August 28). *Consistency is key for weight loss, study says.* CNN. https://edition.cnn.com/2017/08/28/health/weight-loss-consistency-study/index.html

Hughes, L. (2019, December 17). *How does too much sugar affect your body?* WebMD. https://www.webmd.com/diabetes/features/how-sugar-affects-your-body

Hundred Life Design. (2019, March 13). *The importance of consistency in life.* https://hundredlifedesign.com/the-importance-of-consistency-in-life/

Hyman, M. (2014, August 29). *Killing your sex drive one bite at a time: 5 surprising ways sugar lowers libido.* Dr. Mark Hyman. https://drhyman.com/blog/2014/08/29/killing-sex-drive-one-bite-time-5-surprising-ways-sugar-lowers-libido/

Izzy. (2013, February 6). *11 actions you can take today that will drastically improve your health.* Lifehack. https://www.lifehack.org/articles/lifestyle/11-actions-you-can-take-today-that-will-drastically-improve-your-health.html

Jain, V. (2020, May 19). *15 tips to stay consistent on a healthy diet from nutritionist.* NDTV.com. https://www.ndtv.com/health/15-tips-to-stay-consistent-on-healthy-diet-from-nutritionist-2230911

Ketchiff, M. (2018, March 7). *Why consistency is the single most important thing for reaching your health goals.* Shape. https://www.shape.com/weight-loss/tips-plans/consistency-most-important-thing-reach ing-health-goals

Lange, K. (2020, April 16). *Keto fluffy chocolate mousse – 3 ingredients.* The Baking ChocolaTess. https://www.thebakingchocolatess.com/keto-fluffy-chocolate-mousse-3-ingredients/#recipe

Link, R. (2018, September 11). *The 6 best sweeteners on a low-carb keto diet (and 6 to avoid).* Healthline. https://www.healthline.com/nutri tion/keto-sweeteners

Marshall, B. (2018, September 10). *The pros and cons of a keto diet.* Crisp Regional Hospital. https://crispregional.org/the-pros-and-cons-of-a-keto-diet/

Mayo Clinic Staff. (2020, October 8). *Pros and cons of artificial sweeteners.* Mayo Clinic; https://www.mayoclinic.org/healthy-lifestyle/nutrition-and-healthy-eating/in-depth/artificial-sweeteners/art-20046936

McDonell, K., & Kelly, E. (2020, June 4). *9 natural substitutes for sugar.* Healthline; https://www.healthline.com/nutrition/natural-sugar-substitutes

McLintock, K. (2021, April 22). *Sugar detox plan: What to eat during a sugar detox.* Byrdie. https://www.byrdie.com/sugar-detox-recipes

Miller, J. (2016, April 3). *5 steps to removing negative people from your life.* Www.linkedin.com. https://www.linkedin.com/pulse/5-steps-removing-negative-people-from-your-life-joshua-miller/

Montell, A. (2020, June 23). *7 things that happen to your body when you stop eating sugar.* Byrdie. https://www.byrdie.com/stop-eating-sugar

Mucci, K. (2017, January 9). *The illustrated history of how sugar conquered the world.* Saveur. https://www.saveur.com/sugar-history-of-the-world/

Murray, K. (2021, June 15). *Why is sugar addiction a problem?* Addiction-Center. https://www.addictioncenter.com/drugs/sugar-addiction/

Newman, E. (2014, June 30). *Psychology explains why people are so easily duped.* Washington Post. https://www.washingtonpost.com/postev erything/wp/2014/06/30/psychology-explains-why-people-are-so-easily-duped/

Northwestern Medicine Staff. (2019, January 2). *Pros and cons of the ketogenic diet.* Northwestern Medicine. https://www.nm.org/health beat/healthy-tips/nutrition/pros-and-cons-of-ketogenic-diet

Nürnberger, K. (2021, April 26). *Fabulously fudgy keto brownies.* Sugar Free Londoner. https://sugarfreelondoner.com/fabulously-fudgy-keto-brownies/#recipe

OB/GYN Associates of Alabama. (2019, July 26). *12 things that happen when you stop eating sugar.* https://obgynal.com/12-things-that-happen-when-you-stop-eating-sugar/

Oerum, C. (2020, April 19). *Sugar-Free chocolate chip cookies (low-carb).* Diabetes Strong. https://diabetesstrong.com/sugar-free-chocolate-chip-cookies-low-carb/#recipe

Park, W. (2019, May 20). *How your friends change your habits - for better and worse.* Bbc.com. https://www.bbc.com/future/article/20190520-how-your-friends-change-your-habits---for-better-and-worse

Paulas, R. (2015, May 21). *How other people influence your eating.* KCET. https://www.kcet.org/food-discovery/food/how-other-people-influence-your-eating

Pitman, K. R. (n.d.). *Sugar addiction support.* Growing Human(Kind)Ness. Retrieved June 30, 2021, from https://grow inghumankindness.com/sugar-support/

Popik, B. (2010, October 23). *A moment on the lips, forever on the hips.* Www.barrypopik.com. https://www.barrypopik.com/index.php/new_york_city/entry/a_moment_on_the_lips_forever_on_the_hips

Raman, N. (2019, July 16). *5 reasons why consistency is an important habit.* Neelraman.com. https://neelraman.com/5-reasons-why-consis tency-is-an-important-habit/

Rayski, A. (2020, March 3). *9 tasty soda alternatives.* EverydayHealth.-com. https://www.everydayhealth.com/photogallery/soda-alternatives.aspx

Rippe, J., & Angelopoulos, T. (2016). Relationship between added sugars consumption and chronic disease risk factors: Current understanding. *Nutrients*, 8(11), 697. https://doi.org/10.3390/nu8110697

Risher, B. (2021, January 6). *The benefits of a healthy lifestyle*. Healthline. https://www.healthline.com/health/fitness-nutrition/healthy-lifestyle-benefits

Roberts, H. J. (1996). Aspartame as a cause of allergic reactions, including anaphylaxis. *Archives of Internal Medicine*, 156(9), 1027. https://doi.org/10.1001/archinte.1996.00440090139016

Rohn, J. (2016, July 31). *How to deal with the negative influences in your life*. SUCCESS. https://www.success.com/rohn-how-to-deal-with-the-negative-influences-in-your-life/

Satterthwaite, L. (2018, December 11). *The pros and cons of the keto diet*. Promedicahealthconnect.org. https://promedicahealthconnect.org/wellness/the-pros-and-cons-of-the-keto-diet/

Schwecherl, L. (2020, August 13). *30 sugar substitutes for any and every possible situation*. Greatist. https://greatist.com/health/30-sugar-substitutes-any-and-every-possible-situation

Smith, M., Robinson, L., & Segal, J. (2020, September). *Overcoming drug addiction: How to stop abusing drugs, find treatment, and start recovery*. Helpguide.org. https://www.helpguide.org/articles/addictions/overcoming-drug-addiction.htm

Smith, M., Robinson, L., Segal, J., & Segal, R. (2020, September). *Emotional eating and how to stop it*. HelpGuide.org. https://www.helpguide.org/articles/diets/emotional-eating.htm

Solares, A. H. (2021, January 6). *Quit sugar, once and for all*. Fittoserve Group. https://www.fittoservegroup.com/could-i-be-a-sugar-addict/

Stafford, G. (2019, November 11). *The best sugar substitutes for baking & FREE substitutes chart!* Www.biggerbolderbaking.com. https://www.biggerbolderbaking.com/how-to-substitute-sugar/

Stakal, K. (2018, October 22). *Using fruits to replace sugar in your recipes*. Organic Authority. https://www.organicauthority.com/eco-chic-table/using-fruits-to-replace-sugar-in-your-recipes

The Portland Clinic. (2020, January 15). *The keto diet: Pros, cons and tips.* https://www.theportlandclinic.com/the-keto-diet-pros-cons-and-tips/

The Sugar Free Diva. (2020, July 17). *The recipe for delicious sugar free vanilla ice cream.* https://thesugarfreediva.com/sugar-free-vanilla-ice-cream/

U Rock Girl! (2016, December 6). *Baking with sugar substitutes: Which ones are good for baking.* Www.acefitness.org. https://www.acefitness.org/education-and-resources/lifestyle/blog/6193/baking-with-sugar-substitutes-which-ones-are-good-for-baking/

USC Dornsife. (2018, January 30). *Color psychology used in marketing: An overview.* USC MAPP Online. https://appliedpsychologydegree.usc.edu/blog/color-psychology-used-in-marketing-an-overview/

Vitamix. (n.d.). *How to use applesauce as a sugar substitute.* Retrieved July 1, 2021, from https://www.vitamix.com/us/en_us/how-to-use-applesauce-as-a-sugar-substitute

Weil, R. (2021, January 7). Aerobic and anaerobic exercise: Examples and benefits. MedicineNet. https://www.medicinenet.com/aerobic_exercise/article.htm

Zenlama. (2017, November 21). *How to cut negative influences from your life to clear your mind of negativity.* https://www.zenlama.com/how-to-cut-negative-influences-from-your-life-to-clear-your-mind-of-negativity/

Zied, E. (2018, October 17). *5 expert tips to be a healthy influence on others.* SUCCESS. https://www.success.com/5-expert-tips-to-be-a-healthy-influence-on-others/

Printed in Great Britain
by Amazon

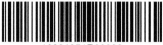

16391951R00092